Recent Results in Cancer Research 145

Managing Editors

P. Schlag, Berlin · H.-J. Senn, St. Gallen

Associate Editors

V. Diehl, Cologne · D.M. Parkin, Lyon
M.F. Rajewsky, Essen · R. Rubens, London
M. Wannenmacher, Heidelberg

Founding Editor

P. Rentchnik, Geneva

Springer
Berlin
Heidelberg
New York
Barcelona
Budapest
Hong Kong
London
Milan
Paris
Santa Clara
Singapore
Tokyo

A. Glaus

Fatigue in Patients with Cancer

Analysis and Assessment

With 16 Figures and 41 Tables

Springer

Agnes Glaus, PhD, MSs, RN

Zentrum für Tumordiagnostik und Prävention
Krebsvorsorge und Pflegeforschung
Rorschacherstr. 150
CH-9007 St. Gallen

ISBN 978-3-642-51468-5 ISBN 978-3-642-51466-1 (eBook)
DOI 10.1007/978-3-642-51466-1

ISSN 0080-0015

Library of Congress Cataloging-in-Publication Data
Glaus, Agnes. Fatigue in patients with cancer: analysis and assessment /A. Glaus. - (Recent results in cancer research, ISSN 0080-0015; 145) Includes bibliographical references and index.
ISBN 978-3-642-51468-5 1. Fatigue - Diagnosis. 2. Cancer - Complications - Diagnosis.
I. Title. II. Series. [DNLM: 1. Neoplasms - complications. 2. Fatigue. W1 RE106P v. 145 1998/QZ 200 G551f 1998] RC261.R35 vol. 145 [RB150.F37] 616.99'4s–dc21 [616.99'4s] DNLM/DLC

Softcover reprint of the hardcover 1st edition 1998

Production: PRO EDIT GmbH, Heidelberg
Typesetting: K+V Fotosatz GmbH, Beerfelden

SPIN 10568335 19/3133-5 4 3 2 1 0 - Printed on acid-free paper

Acknowledgements

This work depends on the contribution of many individuals. I am deeply appreciative of all who made this work possible.

First of all I would like to thank all the patients who were willing to share their fatigue experience in interviews and also patiently filled in the questionnaires. They planted the seed of knowledge about fatigue.

Further I would like to thank my teachers and mentors:

Professor Rosemary Crow, PhD, MA, RGN, SCM, HV, Professor of Nursing at the European Institute of Health and Medical Sciences, University of Guildford, UK, for her continuing scientific and emotional support.

Professor Dr. med. Hans-Jörg Senn, Chairman of the Cancer Center and Head of the Medizinische Klinik C, Kantonsspital St. Gallen, Switzerland, for his encouragement and help in connecting science with clinical relevance.

I would like to thank Dr. Ruedi Maibach and Dr. Jürg Bernhard from the statistical unit and the Quality of Life Office of the Swiss Institute for Applied Cancer Research in Berne for their advice and support in data analyses. I also thank Dr. Sean Hammond, Senior Lecturer at the Department of Psychology, University of Surrey, for his helpful support in the development of the questionnaire.

I would like to thank all my nursing colleagues who were supportive in recruiting and motivating patients to participate in the study, especially Mrs. Christel Böhme, research nurse of the Medizinische Klinik C, Kantonsspital St. Gallen.

Last but not least, I thank my family and friends, who were very patient and supportive throughout this challenging enterprise – with special love to my dear mother and in thankful memory of my father.

Contents

Abstract

Although fatigue is the most frequent complaint in cancer patients, there is no universally accepted definition. In this book a series of studies are presented whose aims were definition of cancer-specific fatigue and the development of an instrument which had the capacity to discriminate levels of fatigue in different groups of cancer patients.

The first study (chapter 2) explored the concept of fatigue by comparing the personal experiences of cancer patients (n=20) with those of healthy individuals (n=20). Using grounded theory, themes emerged which classified fatigue into physical, affective and congitive components. Differences were found in the expressions used by the two cohorts, particularly in relation to the physical sensations experienced. The descriptors generated by cancer patients were compared with those used in the currently available fatigue instruments and illustrated considerable differences in content. They were therefore used to develop a new fatigue instrument – the Fatigue Assessment Questionnaire (FAQ).

The second study (chapter 4) tested the reliability and feasibility of the FAQ in a non-randomised, prospective, cross-sectional study of cancer patients (n=77) and healthy individuals (n=77). It was found to discriminate between fatigue experienced by cancer patients and that experienced by healthy individuals. A tentative step-like theoretical explanation for the production, perception and expression of fatigue proposed at the end of study one was supported by factor analysis. It led to minor adaptations of the instrument.

The third study (chapter 5) subjected the FAQ to further validity testing. Four hundred and ninety-nine cancer patients with a variety of tumour types and stages were included in a prospective, non-randomised, cross-sectional study. Factor analysis supported the theoretical framework and led to modificatons which resulted in a multi-dimensional, 20-item instrument. The FAQ discriminated significantly different levels of fatigue and the distress that it caused in patients with metastatic cancer, patients with localised cancer and patients whose disease was in remission. High levels of fatigue were mainly associated with advanced stages of cancer, in combination with high levels of depression.

The closing chapter represents a synthesis and discusses issues for further research and implications for practice.

The Concept of Fatigue or Tiredness as Experienced in Health and Disease, and More Specifically in Cancer

Fatigue: A General Introduction

In the English and French languages, the word fatigue is used to express feelings of extreme, unusual tiredness. In contrast, Italian-speaking individuals use the word "*stanchezza*" (tiredness) and the German-speaking population also simply uses the word "*Müdigkeit*" (tiredness). The Latin word "*fatigatio*" is translated into German as "general exhaustion" (*allgemeine Erschöpfung*; Duden 1985). The ancient Greeks seem to have felt "*asthenäs*" (strengthless) rather than tired (*kamov/kekmäkos*). In many countries, lay populations would not understand the term fatigue, because there is not even a word for it in their language. In these countries, the term fatigue seems to be replaced by words corresponding to "extreme tiredness" and "general exhaustion."

These linguistic differences reveal the complexity of the concept, which not only represents a semantic problem in different languages and cultures but also raises questions of understanding and interpretation of the phenomenon. Fatigue is a word that is not only used in the context of medicine or psychology; it is also widely used in the technical area of engineering. Material can become fatigued and eventually break down. A similar technical use can be observed in medicine in the phrase fatigue fracture (Reuter and Reuter 1995), a breakdown of bone tissue after exertion.

In *Stedman's Medical Dictionary*, fatigue in humans is "that state following a period of mental or bodily activity characterized by a lessened capacity for work" (Stedman 1973). Even though this definition is of a physiological nature and does not describe how the capacity for work is affected by fatigue, it does point to a concept that is multidimensional in origin. Attempts to define fatigue from a psychological viewpoint require the distinction between fatigue as an objective decrease in performance and general feelings of fatigue which "are not a simple act, but a psychological state made out of a number of simpler elements including changes in affect or sentiments corresponding to obscure and sometimes subconscious tactile and muscular sensations" (Berrios 1990). It seems that the word "fatigue" could be used as an umbrella term to describe a variety of sensations or feelings and expressions of decreased capacity at physical, mental, psychological or social levels. However, no universal definition of fatigue/tiredness as a term used in the context of health and disease is yet available. It is the aim of this chapter to identify fatigue from the viewpoint of health and disease, and specifically from the perspective of cancer.

New Wine in Old Bottles?

Fatigue was already a subject of research in the nineteenth and the early twentieth centuries. Topics of interest from those periods include (Berrios 1990): fatiguability of muscles (Kronecker 1871), the mental symptoms of fatigue (Cowles 1893), questions of "overburdening" (*Ueberbürdungsfrage*; Kraepelin 1898), fatigue from the psychological viewpoint (MacDougall 1899), fatigue measurement in education (Kensies 1898), *fatigue, intellectuel et physique* (fatigue, intellectual and physical; Mosso 1903, in French), a neglected measure of fatigue (Wells 1908), *la fatigue* (Ioteyko 1920, in French), the possibility of a fatigue test (Muscio 1921), fatigue impairment in men (Bartley 1947), and the possibility of treating fatigue (Waterman 1919), among many others. The difficulty of scientific research related to fatigue was expressed by Muscio in 1921, when he recommended "that the term fatigue be absolutely banished from scientific discussion and consequently that attempts to obtain a fatigue test be abandoned" (Muscio 1921). The first scale to measure tiredness was developed during the 1920s (Poffenberger 1928). During the 1960s the first international fatigue conference was organized by Grandjean, a noted fatigue theorist who reviewed neurophysiological experiments to underpin a psychophysiological fatigue theory (Grandjean 1968), together with members of the Japanese Industrial Research Committee on Fatigue, such as Yoshitake, who conducted several studies using his Fatigue Symptom Checklist (Yoshitake 1971). In the 1970s and 1980s the Yoshitake checklist and other scales were used in several nursing studies (Freel and Hart 1977; Haylock and Hart 1979; Davis 1984; Piper et al. 1987). In the meantime, the number of nursing studies on fatigue has increased dramatically. Key publications summarizing the fatigue literature, especially that relating to cancer, have made it easier for nurses to capture the body of present knowledge (Morris 1982; Hart and Freel 1982; Piper et al. 1987; Piper 1993; Irvine and Vincent 1991; Nail and Winningham 1993).

Even though the amount of research and literature has increased dramatically in the last decade, some fundamental questions still prevail. Is tiredness, fatigue or fatiguability more than a single entity, being, in fact, much more a variety of related phenomena? Is fatigue a problem associated with physical processes in the muscles? Is it associated with neurophysiological or psychophysiological processes in the brain or both? What are the causes of unusual tiredness in healthy and in diseased persons?

Physiological or Neurophysiological in Origin?

Fatigue has been described widely in the context of performance of healthy persons at work and in relation to working conditions. The fatigue theorist

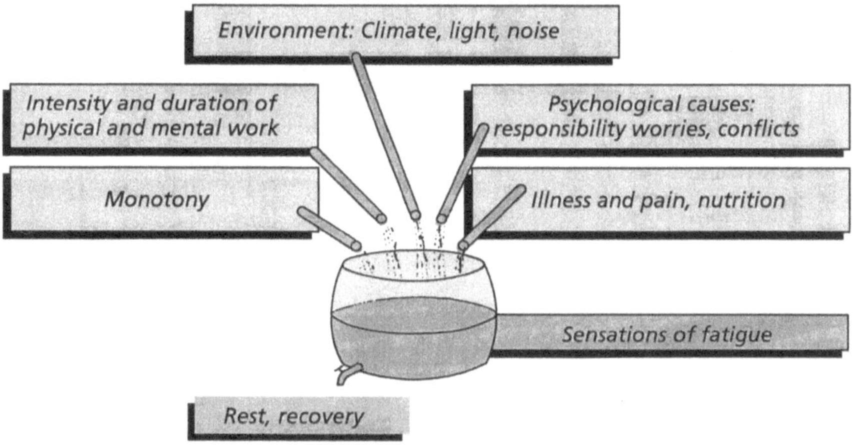

Fig. 1. Cumulative effect of day-to-day causes of fatigue. Based on work by Grandjean (1961)

Grandjean defined it as a pleasant sensation after work, perceived as physiological induction of the sleeping period. He argued that if the body were forced to continue at that point, the sensation would become unpleasant and distressing (Grandjean 1968). Grandjean therefore stressed the biological meaning and aim of tiredness: nature guides the behavior of humans and animals, through feelings of fatigue, to help the body to find its balance between rest and activity. Fatigue in his sense is a life-sustaining state similar to other needs, such as thirst and hunger. However, experts agree that there is a need for delineation between different words in the attempt to define fatigue. Physiology distinguishes between muscle fatigue and general fatigue. Muscle fatigue is described as local, acute fatigue induced by exertion. General fatigue is seen as a state in which humans perceive tiredness as reduced performance, and Grandjean also defined this state as general, mental or nervous fatiguability. He attempted to identify the causes of fatiguability in healthy persons from the physiologist's viewpoint; these causes are illustrated in Fig. 1 (translated from German): the diverse, daily sensations of fatigue accumulate until the body stops functioning and recovery allows draining of these sensations to take place (Grandjean 1961).

Grandjean interprets physiological fatigue as a decrease in physical performance, but also as a consequence of neurophysiological processes. Experiments with continuous electrical stimulation of the midbrain, especially the thalamus, in cats resulted in sedation, with reduced reaction and a tendency to sleep (Hess 1948; Akert and Koella 1952). On the basis of these findings, Grandjean suggested that structures in the midbrain might represent an active inhibitory system. Cortical inhibition may result from two different causes: cortical activity may be reduced by increased activity of the inhibitory system, which appears to be regulated through humoral factors. Secondly, the reticular activating system (RAS) in the midline of the brain stem, which is known to be responsible for maintaining wakefulness and alerting the cortex, appears to effect feelings of fatigue through secretion and accumulation of serotonin. Grandjean labels this process the active inhibitory system. When the RAS is inhibited, the organism is in a state of fatigue; if the activating system prevails, the organism is ready to increase performance and feels fresh and full of initiative. In the light of present neurophysiological knowledge, generalized fatigue could be considered a central nervous system state controlled by antagonistic activity of inhibitory and activating systems of the brain stem (Hart and Freel 1982).

A Human Response Designed to Maintain Health?

In general, fatigue is frequently regarded as something to be avoided. Avoidance of fatigue may not be entirely desirable if it is viewed in relation to the process of adaptation needed to maintain health. Fatigue sensations may be essential indicators that the physiological equilibrium somewhere in the body is breaking down (Dill 1967). It can be an index of stress on adaptive mechanisms. Therefore, fatigue could be defined as a defense mechanism, a protective phenomenon that helps to maintain physiological equilibrium by stimulating a desire for work decrements or stress avoidance when the response to stress reaches a level of discomfort (Bartley 1967). It could be argued, however, that the wish to do work or to avoid stress may have roots other than fatigue.

Deviations from "normal" tiredness are not always easy to recognize. The activity of the human organism is rhythmical and geared toward the maintenance of a dynamic, healthy equilibrium. Well-known processes, such as circadian rhythms, cardiac work–rest cycles, humoral and neural balances and compensatory mechanisms, all contribute to maintaining this dynamic equilibrium. In health, the body is not only rhythmical in function but is also maintained in a state of watchfulness. The state of slight muscle contraction, the ease with which flight–fight forces are initiated, and the so-called conservation withdrawal process, which warns of impending energy depletion, are normal reactions that enable the organism to maintain a balanced state in spite of constant bombardment from internal and external stimuli (Morris 1982). This ability to adapt has been described as "human adaptation capacity," the individual's ability to cope successfully with the stresses of life – a capacity encompassing the morphological, biological, chemical, physiological and psychological processes that bring about coping responses (Bafitis and Sargent 1977). Tiredness, which is seen as a regulative, protective mechanism, could be called healthy tiredness. "Acceptable" fatigue includes recognition of tiredness and steps taken to overcome it as soon as possible, enabling the person to sustain performance. Persons who are able to sustain performance perceive themselves as healthily tired; their tiredness does not make them anxious (Nixon 1976).

This definition of healthy tiredness has some similarity with the general definition of health given by Dubos (1959), who defines health as the ability to adapt. Adaptation in his sense does not necessarily mean living without disease, but rather being able to live with disease. It has been postulated that in healthy persons increasing arousal results in increasing performance and that persisting arousal without performance would lead to deterioration, breakdown and ill health (Nixon 1976). This would mean that fatigue can be seen as a protective mechanism designed to maintain health and to prevent illness. On the other hand, fatigue or unusual tiredness can mean the person affected has successfully fought off critical situations or conditions, or is on the road to recovery. Clinical experience shows that after serious illness or after major surgery patients experience extreme feelings of tiredness. This could be interpreted as fatigue or tiredness that has to be experienced in order to regain health. Whether this kind of fatigue, again, represents a protective mechanism and whether it is physiological or psychological in nature is difficult to distinguish. It could, however, be concluded that people need tiredness to maintain health, to prevent illness, and/or to regain health. The degree to which a person should respond to that tiredness must be seen as a matter of individual needs and resources, because health, defined as the ability to adapt, represents an individual challenge as well.

Are There Vulnerable Populations?

People generally believe that age plays a part in relation to fatigue, attributing higher levels of fatigue to the older population. Data from a large survey (n=2000) of American adults between 25 and 74 years of age were used to explore the relationship of self-perceived fatigue and age, gender, body mass, nutritional intake, activity and emotional distress (Chen 1986). Chen concluded from his study that there was no association between age and fatigue. A newer study, examining fatigue in general practice attendees, concluded that there was no correlation between age and the total fatigue scores for men and women (David and Pelosi 1990). A further study, comparing fatigue between 104 breast cancer patients and 93 healthy women, did not describe differences in age in the control group (Irvine and Vincent 1994). Few fatigue studies have included a control group with healthy individuals. Methodological problems in defining and measuring fatigue make it difficult to interpret and compare results.

Gender has been defined by Chen (1986) as a risk factor. He concluded that in women the risk of being fatigued was 1.5 times the risk in men. David found no difference between men and women in his study (David and Pelosi 1990), and Glaus (1993) found higher mean levels of fatigue in women than in men.

Chen found no difference for any nutrient in the diet between nonfatigued and fatigued women. The only significant difference between fatigued and nonfatigued men was a higher calcium intake in the nonfatigued men. Difficulties arising from potentially confounding variables have been discussed. Body mass was not found to be a significant predictor of fatigue. Chen's study supports the influence of activity on fatigue. Inactive subjects had more than twice the risk of those who were active of being afflicted with fatigue. He also reported a significant association of self-perceived fatigue with psychological factors, such as depression, emotional stress and anxiety (Chen 1986).

A Response to Disease?

Fatigue has been described as a warning signal of an approaching health disaster (Morris 1982). As an example, excessive tiredness may precede 30%–55% of myocardial infarctions and sudden cardiac deaths (Appels and Mulder 1988). General fatigue in patients with cardiac disease might be due to the failure of circulatory and metabolic adaptations, such as increased cardiac output or decreased efficiency of oxygen transport (Hart and Freel 1982). The same can be said for patients with lung disease or persistent anemia. This kind of fatigue might be classified as "caused by circulatory and metabolic adaptation failure."

Fatigue has also been identified as one of the top three stressors experienced by hemodialysis and peritoneal dialysis patients (Eichel 1986). Srivastava (1989) studied characteristics of the fatigue experience in end-stage renal disease patients. Although hemodialysis improved their well-being tremendously once the treatment was initiated, complaints about fatigue generally continued. Srivastava concluded that even though the toxic effect of uremia with low levels of hemoglobin could be responsible for fatigue in these patients, the components of the symptom remained unknown and seemed rather to be physiological and nonspecific. Fatigue associated with renal disease could be classified as fatigue caused by metabolic disorders. However, other researchers have shown that depression can go hand in hand with chronic disease, such as chronic renal disease, and that psychological components of fatigue should be assessed as well as physiological ones (Cardenas and Kutner 1982).

Patients suffering from multiple sclerosis identified fatigue as their most troublesome symptom (Krupp and Alvarez 1988). A study of patients with rheumatoid arthritis highlighted the prevalence of fatigue: 52% of 101 patients stated that they constantly lacked energy (Crosby 1991). Whether fatigue in these conditions could be classified as primarily caused by immunological processes remains to be substantiated. Fatigue and muscular weakness are also prevalent symptoms in patients with primary hyperparathyroidism. The improvement in muscle strength could be documented in a controlled study in which patients were treated by surgical parathyroidectomy with correction of hypercalcaemia (Kristoffersson and Boström 1992). Addison's disease is known to be accompanied by weakness and easy fatiguability. These two conditions might be two examples of diseases that are "caused by endocrine disturbances." However, in all these severe disease states, influences of such physical and psychological effects of chronic illness as changes in activity, sleep disturbance, pain, and emotional distress cannot be excluded.

It has been suggested that fatigue in patients with AIDS was more severe than in patients with bone marrow transplantation or malignant melanoma (Fawzy and Cousin 1990). Clinical experience shows that fatigue is a universal complaint in AIDS. Whether this kind of fatigue can be classified as primarily caused by immunological or neurological processes has not yet been defined.

The chronic fatigue syndrome (CFS) has recently received a great deal of attention from the media and from health care professionals alike. It has also been labeled a postviral syndrome, because the symptoms often follow an illness suggestive of viral infection (Behan and Behan 1985), or myalgic encephalomyelitis (ME). It has been argued that these last two descriptors are inappropriate, first because a defined initiating infection was not always documented and patients with CFS reported an insidious onset, and secondly because myalgia was not universal among patients and no laboratory tests showed evidence of encephalitis or myelitis. The diagnosis is now defined by the following criteria: (a) generalized, chronic fatigue over 6 months in duration, (b) neuropsychiatric dysfunction (impairment of concentration, short-term memory impairment) and (c) abnormal cell-mediated immunity resulting from reduction of lymphocyte subsets (T8 and/or T4). Further supporting findings are myalgia, arthralgia, headaches, depression, tinnitus, paresthesia and sleep disturbance, persistence for over 6 months with no other cause, and lymphadenopathy, localized muscle tenderness and pharyngitis on two or more occasions after the illness (Lloyd and Wakefield 1988). The exclusion of any other clinical disease is part of the diagnosis. It is still not clear whether CFS is caused primarily by viral infections or disorders of the immune system and whether endocrine and psychological causes have any role in it (Siegl 1994). Because CFS was seen as an organic diagnosis that included psychiatric features, it remained unclear what diagnosis would be assigned to patients known to have psychiatric syndromes identified in the *Diagnostic and Statistical Manual of Mental Disorders*, 3rd edition, revised (DSM III-R; Greenberg 1990). The classification of causes therefore remains difficult.

Rooted in Body or Mind?

CFS has stirred up a lot of discussion about the roots of fatigue. Several researchers have acknowledged that psychiatric disorders, particularly mood disorders, are common in patients with chronic fatigue (Greenberg 1990). Are these patients ill because they are depressed or are they depressed because they are ill? The terms "neurasthenia," "brain fatigue," "psychasthenia," "adynamia," "anxiety neurosis," and "neurotic fatigue" (Greenberg 1990), which were used in different epochs, point to the many-sided interpretation of the symptom of chronic fatigue. In truth, the syndrome falls through the

Table 1. Causes of fatigue: primary impact of disorders associated with specific disease

Disorder	Associated diseases
Circulatory and metabolic adaptation failure (decreased oxygen carrying capacity)	Heart, lung disease Severe anemia Cancer
Metabolic disorders (hypercalcaemia, hyponatremia, hypoglycemia)	Renal disease, uremia Liver disease Hyperparathyroidism Cancer
Endocrine, hormonal disturbances	Addison's disease Disease of pituitary and adrenal glands Parathyroid disease Cancer
Disruption of central nervous functions	Brain disease Cancer
Chronic infections and humoral disorders	AIDS Chronic fatigue syndrome? Viral infections? Cancer?
Immunological, auto-immune processes	Rheumatoid arthritis Multiple sclerosis Cancer?
Emotional distress associated with chronic disease	Any chronic disease

net between a number of medical specialties, including medicine and psychiatry. Many people consider a psychiatric diagnosis to be a stigma and might therefore prefer to have a viral infection identified as the cause.

The link between sadness and fatigue has already been confirmed many times. Engel and Schmale (1972) saw helplessness and hopelessness as central to the conservation withdrawal reaction, which they connected with the constitutional symptom of fatigue. Although few studies have acknowledged that fatigue makes any distinct contribution to the syndrome of major depression, it remains one of the identified criteria allowing a diagnosis of clinical depression (Nelson and Charney 1981). There appears to be a lack of data arising out of sound research to underpin the relationship between fatigue and depression, even though this relationship seems to be a generally accepted fact. Greenberg (1990) noted that 90% of patients with depression reported decreased energy. One typical sign of tiredness in depression, as shown by clinical experience, might be its worsening in the mornings. This typical sign could distinguish this type of tiredness from the tiredness associated with other illnesses, but this notion remains to be substantiated.

Anxiety has been seen as a correlate of fatigue. In a study among college students who complained of excessive fatigue the symptom of anxiety was common, and they also had higher scores on the Beck Depression Inventory than did control subjects (Montgomery 1983). Anxiety could be seen as forerunner of or concomitant with fatigue. If the anxious state is relieved, a conservation withdrawal process can result (Morris 1982), leading to feelings of tiredness and depression. Further research is needed to test such hypotheses. A summary of the primary causes of fatigue in humans is presented in Table 1.

Fatigue and Cancer: Inevitable Twins?

Priority and Prevalence

Fatigue in cancer patients was ranked as a major concern in the American Oncology Nursing Society Research Priority Surveys of 1991 (Mooney et al. 1991) and also of 1994 (Stetz et al. 1994). A fatigue initiative was started in 1994, and the American Oncology Nursing Society set out to develop a plan for dissemination of information on fatigue. From that, the FIRE Program (Fatigue Initiative through Research and Education) originated, with research and education as the program's primary focus (ONS News 1996).

Today, fatigue is recognized as the most common and perhaps the most distressing symptom reported by cancer patients. Owing to methodological problems in defining and measuring fatigue in cancer patients, figures on the exact prevalence of tiredness in patients with different types of malignant tumors or with different treatment schedules are scarce and difficult to compare (McCorkle and Quint-Benoliel 1983; Piper and Lindsey 1989; World Health Organisation 1990; Blesch and Paice 1991; Butow and Coates 1991; Holmes 1991; Glaus 1993). More insight has been gained into the incidence of fatigue as a treatment side effect during the last 10 years, and especially since treatment entered the era of biological response modifiers (Haylock and Hart 1979; Jamar 1982; Bruera 1988; Piper and Rieger 1989; Irvine and Vincent 1994). The lack of proven therapeutic strategies to relieve this distressing symptom underscores the need for future research with an internationally agreed definition and with validated measurement instruments for epidemiological fatigue research.

Etiology of Fatigue in Cancer

Individuals with cancer might experience different types of fatigue or tiredness. They can experience acute tiredness as a consequence of exertion or performance at work, as healthy individuals do, although they might be more vulnerable to fatiguability during active disease. This type of tiredness might be acute tiredness localized primarily in specific muscle groups and be temporary and resolved by rest and time. Clinical experience indicates that chronic fatigue in cancer patients, as it is conceived of here, lasts more than 2 weeks and has a recurring character, is mostly not associated with ex-

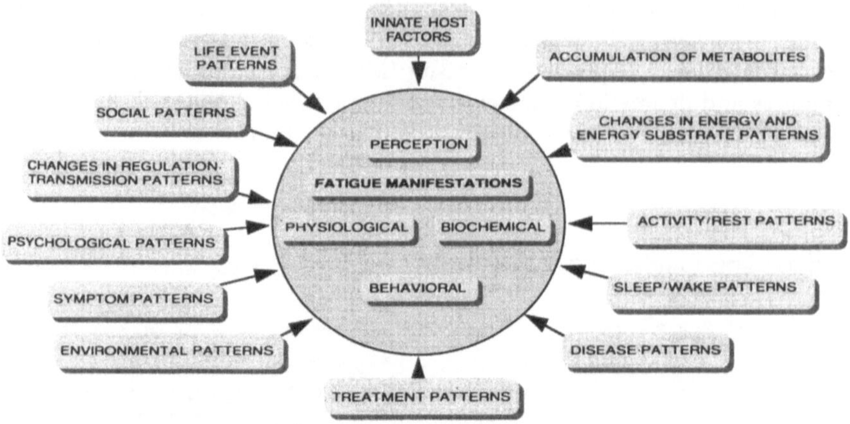

Fig. 2. Piper's integrated fatigue model. Based on work by Piper et al. (1987)

ertion but represents a general fatigue state affecting the whole person in body and mind. Even though objective fatigue is often reported as a decrease in strength and performance by severely ill cancer patients and might also be observable by others, the subjective feelings of fatigue remain difficult to analyze and to assess, although they might have a severely negative impact on the quality of life. The relationship between tiredness as experienced by healthy individuals and tiredness as experienced by cancer patients needs further research in order to delineate specific features in patients with cancer.

Although some theoretical models have evolved in the last decade to explain fatigue in cancer patients, none of them could be tested scientifically (Piper 1993; Winningham and Nail 1994). The most frequently cited theoretical framework on fatigue in cancer is that developed by Piper et al. (1987), which is presented in Fig. 2. This model addresses many potential causes of fatigue in cancer and stresses the multidimensionality of the concept. The impressive diversity of possibly confounding influences represents the complex reality, and researchers need to break down and weight the elements to test relevant, specific hypotheses in a scientific manner.

Fatigue Caused by the Primary Impact of Cancer on the Affected Organs

The primary pathophysiological causes of fatigue in humans, as presented in Table 1, are the same in cancer patients. According to the infiltration of the primary tumor or its metastatic spread, disturbances of the physiological system might follow. If pulmonary or cardiac function is insufficient as a result of local tumor mass, additional infection or severe anemia, fatigue is caused by a decreased circulatory capacity for oxygen supply. If the tumor impairs renal or hepatic function, fatigue might be caused by metabolic disorders. Cancerous destruction of locations of the hormonal system, such as adrenal glands or the pituitary gland, may lead to fatigue by way of hormonal endocrine dysfunction with metabolic complications (Morant 1991). Tumor infiltration of the brain can lead to fatigue caused directly by increased cerebral pressure or destruction of central nervous functions. Many types of cancer, especially those of the lymphatic and blood-producing systems, can lead to fatigue by way of humoral deficiencies, with decreased defense mechanisms and a predisposition to frequent infections and bleeding.

Fatigue caused by the immunological responses to the tumor and fatigue caused by the psychological demands arising from illness have a special place in the development of fatigue in cancer, and therefore these causes will be discussed in more detail later.

Fatigue Caused by Secondary Effects of Cancer

Asthenins

Apart from the many direct primary causes of fatigue produced by the local changes arising from tumor infiltration, there are other, secondary paraneoplastic pathways, a summary of which is presented in Table 2. It has been proposed that the malignant process itself may secrete substances, also called "asthenins," that cause asthenia (Theologides 1982). Asthenia, in this sense, has been defined as pathologic fatiguability, loss of strength and generalized weakness (Bruera 1988) and can thus be seen as a major component of fatigue as defined earlier. Such asthenins are substances that cause morphological, biochemical or physiological changes in tumor-free muscle tissue in cancer patients. These changes in the muscles are thought to be the causes of asthenia (Theologides 1986). In cancer patients with advanced disease, abnormal electrophysiological changes in the muscles can be observed, which are independent of malnutrition and loss of muscle tissue (Bruera and Bremmeis 1988). While it is still unclear whether these asthenins are produced by the tumor or by the immune system, it is also unclear whether the muscle changes are responsible for asthenia or whether they represent an epiphenomenon (Stiefel and Morant 1992). Muscle wasting occurring in the course of advanced cancer was thought to be responsible for fatigue, because it requires patients to exert an unusually high amount of effort to generate adequate contractile force and changed muscular metabolism may occur (St. Pierre and Kaspar 1992).

Side Effect of the Body's Response to the Tumor?

A further proposed definition of fatigue is "the body's inflammatory defense mechanism against the tumor," analogous to the situation in infectious disease. The secretion of cytokines, such as interferons, interleukins and tumor necrosis factors by monocytes and inflammatory cells activated in response

Table 2. Causes of fatigue: secondary impact of cancer on body and mind

Cancer-related, secondary causes	Effects
Cytokines	Defense mechanisms against the tumor
"Asthenins"	Changes in muscle metabolism Muscle wasting
Cachexins	Change in energy transformation
Interferons, interleukins	Impairment of protein synthesis
Tumor necrosis factor	Weight loss Delayed gastric emptying
Increased energy expenditure	Increased muscle protein loss Increased effort to generate force Increased metabolism Increased fat mobilization Decreased food intake
Paraneoplastic syndromes	Hypercalcemia, hyponatremia Hypoglycemia
Other symptoms of disease	Immobility, sleep disturbance, pain and others
Emotional distress, coping	Depression, anxiety, social isolation
Cancer treatment (chemotherapy, radiotherapy, biotherapy, surgery)	Accumulation of waste products? Reaction to necrotic tissue from cell breakdown? Temporary organ toxicity Side effects (nausea/emesis/anorexia) Immobility? inactivity? Central neurophysiological mechanisms Deficit of vitamins and nutrients during increased demands? Tissue damage and healing

to the neoplastic process involves a whole cascade of reactions, and fatigue and associated phenomena may be expected to be caused by this underlying process (Morant 1991). However, not all tumor types activate the immune system, and some might even cause immune suppression.

Chronic stimulation by endogenous interferon-γ can be measured as elevated neopterin levels indicating activated macrophages. Decreased levels of tryptophan associated with increased neopterin levels may impair protein synthesis and may be a defense mechanism against the active proliferation of tumors (Denz and Orth 1993). Tryptophan is a precursor substance of serotonin, which has also been used as sleep medication. A tiring effect could be expected from such a substance.

Endogenous tumor necrosis factor (TNF) leads, as the word suggests, to tumor necrosis, but also to protein degradation, weight and muscle loss, and anorexia (Beutler and Cerami 1987). Some TNFs are secreted primarily by macrophages and monocytes, but they may also be produced by various tumor cells (Naylor and Malik 1990). A second (earlier) name for TNF is cachexin, which describes its devastating effects. Cachexia might be due to central effects of TNF but could also be due to delayed gastric emptying (Bodnar and Pasternak 1989).

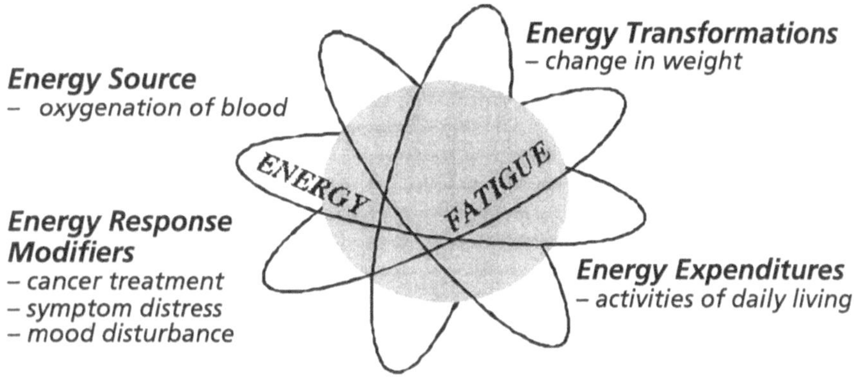

Fig. 3. Energy analysis model. Based on work by Irvine and Vincent (1994)

Energy Transformation Processes in Cancer

Patients with advanced cancer and cachexia typically demonstrate modestly increased rates of energy expenditure in the presence of diminished food intake owing to anorexia and to gastrointestinal disturbances (Keller 1993). Rates of glucose production by the liver, gluconeogenesis and glycolysis yielding lactate metabolism are increased, and fat mobilization and oxidation are accelerated. A redistribution of body proteins away from muscle towards visceral proteins, resulting in marked muscle protein loss, can be observed (Keller 1993). The loss of muscle tissue caused by this mechanism might be responsible for muscle weakness, which requires patients to exert an unusually large amount of effort to generate adequate contractile force, as discussed above. The energy analysis model in the context of fatigue in cancer patients (Fig. 3) offered by Irvine and Vincent (1994) takes account of these changes in energy transformation processes. The interaction of energy variables, such as sources, transformation and expenditure, and characteristics such as weight loss, fatigue and activity intolerance are discussed in the model. It can be suggested that changes in energy sources, transformation and expenditure might be far too complex to be limited to oxygenation and changes in weight and in activities of daily living. Energy intake might also be influenced by resorption or digestion; transformation and expenditure of energy might also be influenced by complex, biochemical and immunological processes.

Conflicting results have been reported by Bruera and Brenneis (1989), who did not find any correlation between nutritional status, lean body mass, tumor mass, anemia, type of treatment and asthenia scores in a study of patients with locally recurrent or metastatic breast cancer. The only positive correlation was found between asthenia scores and depression. It remains to be tested whether there is an association between these variables in patients with other types of cancer. With reference to body weight, a study of weight loss in cancer patients showed that the least weight loss was experienced by patients with breast cancer, with gastric cancer patients experiencing the most pronounced losses of weight (De Wys and Begg 1980). It could be hypothesized that different types and stages of cancer are associated with different amounts and types of cytokine production, which goes hand in hand with tumor activity and its devastating consequences, one of which is weakness and fatigue.

Paraneoplastic Syndromes

Paraneoplastic syndromes, which might induce fatigue, are known in some types of cancer. Secretions of mediators by the tumor, such as parathormone-related factors, antidiuretic hormone and similar substances, may have severe metabolic consequences, such as hypercalcemia, hyponatremia, and hypoglycemia, all of which may cause fatigue. Hypercalcemia induced by active osteolytic substances is frequently seen in patients with skeletal metastasis of breast cancer and in patients with non-small-cell lung cancer. This frequently seen secondary disease can lead to muscular weakness, fatigue, dehydration, hyporeflexia and further symptoms (Senn and Drings 1992).

Association with Cancer Treatment

Surgery

The problem of postoperative fatigue is not well understood. Clinical experience shows that it improves with time. It is unclear whether it is a consequence of tissue damage and healing, or whether it results from deconditioning because of immobility. Postoperative pain medication and nutritional demands may also have a role. Depending on the type of surgery, the patient is confronted with changes of body image and function and needs energy to adapt to new conditions. If surgery leads to the identification of a diagnosis of cancer, psychological distress, such as anxiety and depression, might lead to a fatigued condition (Christensen and Hjortso 1986).

Radiotherapy

Destruction of tumor cells by irradiation is an unusual condition for the body, which is left with the elimination of waste products. Cell damage and the reaction of the body to necrotic tissue have been discussed in the context of fatigue in radiotherapy patients. Although it is common today to attribute fatigue in patients with radiotherapy to the production of by-products of cell death, little is known to underpin this belief.

Side effects of radiotherapy are usually localized, based on the site of treatment. Fatigue is one of the few systemic side effects and has been found to increase towards the end of treatment (Haylock and Hart 1979; King and Nail 1985). A decrease of fatigue during the pauses at weekends was observed in a study by Haylock and Hart (1979), who measured fatigue with the Pearson-Byars Fatigue Checklist. Contradictory findings have been reported from a study by Nail and Winningham (1993), who found that fatigue did not decrease over the weekend in pretreated or posttreated women undergoing intracavitary radiation therapy for gynecological cancer. King and Nail (1985) interviewed 96 radiotherapy patients and found that they perceived fatigue as intermittent early in treatment but that it became a continuous state by the end of treatment and was worse in the afternoon or evening. King also observed higher fatigue levels before radiotherapy in patients with lung cancer than in patients with other cancer diagnoses. Somnolence was found in 100% of patients receiving cranial irradiation (Faithfull 1991). It can be argued that somnolence in this condition either reflects cognitive impairment through cerebral edema or is caused by the cerebral disease itself, rather than being caused by irradiation.

These and further studies in radiotherapy patients have led to the generation of the following speculations: (1) Fatigue levels correlate primarily with characteristics of the disease: fatigue levels of patients with lung cancer might primarily be different from fatigue levels in breast or gynecological cancer. (2) The type and aim of radiotherapy, for example adjuvant in breast cancer or palliative in lung cancer, have an important role. (3) Successful radiotherapy could relieve fatigue if it ameliorates the function of a specific organ, such as the lung, by successfully decreasing tumor size and increasing the breathing capacity. (4) Adjuvant irradiation, for example after breast surgery, does not increase any organ function or relieve distress, but is perceived as an additional, fatiguing burden. These and many more questions deserve further investigation.

Chemotherapy

As in the case of radiotherapy, the mechanisms of fatigue development are poorly understood in the context of chemotherapy treatment. Cell damage and reactions to cell necrosis are, again, generally accepted explanations. In contrast to the usually localized effect of radiotherapy, chemotherapeutic cancer treatment, according to its type and intensity, might damage healthy cells as well as cancer cells everywhere in the body. This generalized influence on the whole body system might explain chemotherapy's severe impact. In many studies, fatigue has been demonstrated to be the most prevalent side effect in patients receiving chemotherapy (Knoff 1986; Nerenz and Leventhal 1982; Meyerowitz and Watkins 1983; Rhodes and Watson 1988; Bloom and Gorsky 1990; Blesch and Paice 1991). A hypothesis emerging on this point is that chemotherapeutic agents can theoretically reach cells of all organs and therefore have the potential to induce fatigue by effects on every organ and in this way can produce general fatigue as well as "organ-specific fatigue reactions," according to the specific target. This includes the hypothesis that the various cytotoxic drugs affect different organs in different ways.

Chemotherapy patients often relate fatigue directly to their treatment, and clinical experience shows that they exhibit increased energy just before the next therapy cycle. Intensity and duration are perceived differently by individuals and might be correlated with regimen and type of drugs. Richardson (1996) investigated the onset, pattern, duration, intensity and distress associated with fatigue in chemotherapy patients. Data indicated that although fatigue may be essentially similar among groups receiving different chemotherapy regimens, there is significant individual variation in its severity and the amount of associated distress. An increase in distress has been noted with progression of therapy (Love and Leventhal 1989) in a descriptive study of patients with ovarian cancer, which documented the fatigue trajectory through a chemotherapy cycle. Love and Leventhal's study gave researchers a helpful lesson: no difference was found between the patients and healthy individuals. The explanation for this unexpected finding was the timing of the measurement of fatigue used to compare the groups, as it did not capture the occurrence of fatigue. Methodological aspects of measurement, such as timing, are potential biases, especially in chemotherapy patients.

Cytotoxic drugs might be the primary cause of fatigue in these patients, although a variety of other influences need to be analyzed. Other side effects of treatment, such as nausea, emesis, decrease of nutritional intake, unusual anemia, could be linked with higher fatigue levels. Antiemetic drugs, especially sedating substances, are expected to increase fatigue. These influences are supported by the clinical experience that fatigue in chemotherapy patients is most prominent during and for some days after treatment. The hypothesis is often heard that fatigue correlates with the time of the blood cell nadir; but this needs verification.

The four hypotheses formulated to explain fatigue in the context of radiation therapy (above) can all be formulated in the context of chemotherapy in cancer patients or in the context of combined treatment. The same basic questions remain to be answered.

Biotherapy

In addition to the potential mechanisms for treatment-related fatigue as described earlier, biotherapy exposes patients to exogenous and endogenous cytokines. Interferons, interleukin-2, TNFs and colony-stimulating factors are the substances most often used in cancer treatment. Biotherapy-related fatigue usually becomes manifest as part of a syndrome, the so-called flu-like syndrome, involving fatigue, fever, chills, myalgia, headache and malaise (Haeuber 1989). Fatigue has been seen as a dose-limiting factor in treatment with biotherapy (Piper and Rieger 1989). Cognitive deficits, such as the expression of mental fatigue, have been associated with biotherapy side effects. In a study with ten interferon-treated cancer patients, neuropsychiatric investigations revealed a lack of energy and reduced motivation to initiate activities. The cognitive and affective impairment observed was similar to the symptoms found in patients with pathologic processes in the frontal lobe

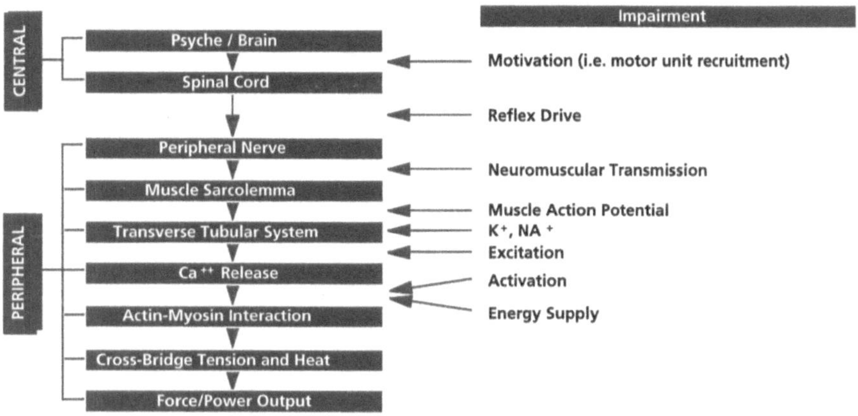

Fig. 4. Central and peripheral mechanisms of fatigue. Based on work by Gibson and Edwards (1989)

(Adams and Queseda 1984), and it was therefore concluded that patients who received interferon therapy had experienced toxicity of the frontal lobe. The central mechanisms are thought to hold the possible key to the explanation of fatigue in biotherapy patients. The theoretical framework developed by Gibson and Edwards (1985) to define central and peripheral neurophysiological mechanisms of fatigue, gives support to this type of fatigue (Fig. 4). The central mechanisms may include impaired spinal cord transmission, or recruitment of motor neurons (Piper and Rieger 1989) or "an exhaustion or malfunctioning of brain cells in the hypothalamic region" (Poteliakhoff 1981).

Social and psychological adaptation to disease and to the demands of treatment are thought to have a major influence in radiotherapy as well as in chemotherapy and biotherapy. The need for more rest, as clinically seen in many patients, requires adaptation of the working schedule. Some patients may prefer to interrupt work for certain periods or to reduce it. If therapy comes into patients' lives as an extra time-consuming factor, in addition to their usual work, it could be hypothesized that fatigue will be an outcome of overexertion. Aspects of fatigue and its relationship with anxiety and depression in the context of coping with cancer will be addressed later.

Other Symptoms Arising from Cancer and Its Treatment

Fatigue has been assigned a unique position relative to other symptoms by Winningham and Nail (1994), based on its effect on activity and functional status (Fig. 5). Cancer patients are thought to become less active as a result of symptoms such as pain, nausea/vomiting, dyspnea, diarrhea, fever, anxiety, depression, and fatigue, resulting in a loss of energizing metabolic resources. The outcome of decreased activity is described as secondary fatigue

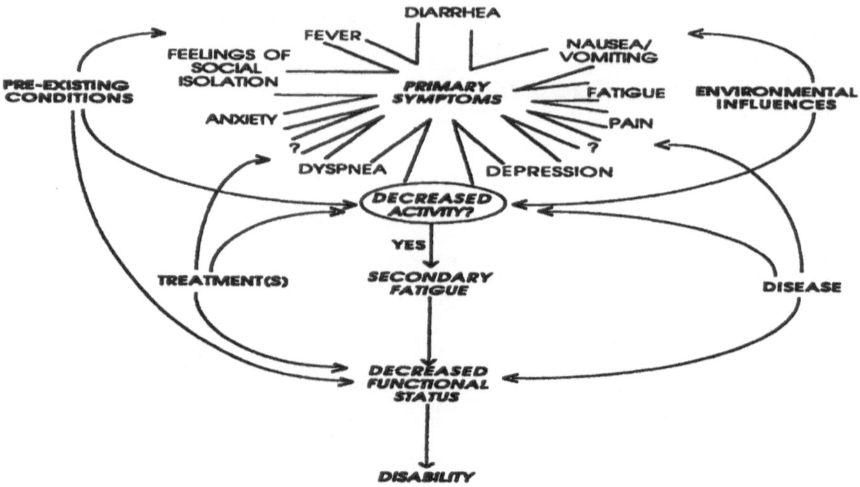

Fig. 5. Winningham's psychobiological entropy model. Based on work by Winningham and Nail (1994)

attributable to decreased energetic capacity (oxygen uptake, calorie consumption) leading to reduced functional status. Symptoms that induce more rest and inactivity might lead to secondary fatigue, but also require treatments that could induce fatigue. Medications, such as antiemetic substances and pain and sleep medications, are known to have potential fatiguing effects. Conflicting findings make it difficult to know whether anemia itself can be a direct cause of fatigue. If anemia is severe and causes inactivity, then secondary fatigue could the consequence of reduced activity. In the light of Winningham's theory, immobilization could be a fatigue-inducing state. This framework represents a challenge for the nursing profession, as mobility is an important concept in nursing care. However important the influence of activity and functional status on fatigue might be, it needs to be seen in the context of the primary and secondary causes of fatigue in cancer, as summarized in Tables 1 and 2.

Cancer, Coping, Anxiety, and Depression

Coping with cancer means dealing with a reality that healthy persons usually deny. If cancer, usually seen as a disease "of others," happening to others, suddenly happens in one's own life, the fragility of life can no longer be denied. The existential outlook of a person affected with a potentially mortal disease may require him or her to withdraw to enable coping, and fatigue may be a coping mechanism, expressed as a feeling of depression. There is no scientific evidence to support the hypothesis, but it is generally accepted that depressed persons report chronic fatigue. Greenberg (1990) noted that 90% of patients with depression reported decreased energy and that fatigue remained a criterion of the diagnosis of clinical depression. The validated instrument POMS (Profile of Mood States), with which mood disturbances are assessed, includes a subscale to assess vigor and fatigue (McNair and Lorr 1971). Weisman (1979) described various meanings of "I feel very tired all the time" and notes that long drawn-out fatigue is both a cause and a symptom of emotional distress.

In cancer patients, it seems important to distinguish between depression and fatigue, because different treatment approaches might be needed. It is difficult to rely on the results of existing studies because different measurement instruments have been used in different populations, resulting in both positive (Jamar 1982; Bruera and Brenneis 1989; Piper and Lindsey 1989; Blesch and Paice 1991) and negative correlations (Srivastava 1989; Pickard-Holley 1991). It can be argued that feeling sad and depressed is a reaction to the whole life-threatening situation of a cancer patient and that tiredness results from the body's attempt to deal with disease, treatment and its consequences rather than being an expression of fatigue itself. In this sense, tiredness could be seen as a symptom of coping and depression. On the other hand, there is evidence for physical causes of tiredness in cancer patients, as described earlier. The question of whether tiredness is a symptom of disease or a symptom of coping and depression, or whether it is a combination of both, remains unanswered. It can be hypothesized that these two potential sources of tiredness should be seen as a differential diagnosis needing careful assessment and different treatment approaches. Consideration of patient history, such as psychological difficulties in the past, social vulnerability, such as social isolation and lack of a supporting network, as well as disease-specific influences, such as brain tumor lesions or metabolic disorders, seem crucial in diagnosing the causes of tiredness.

Anxiety, which is known to prepare humans for danger, has been described as a forerunner of and concomitant with fatigue (Morris 1982). The relief of an anxious state might result in a depressive state, or a failure to resolve causes of the anxious state might lead to exhaustion. Clinical experience shows that cancer disease and its treatment can be sources of intensive anxiety over long periods of time. An interesting observation described by Simms and Rhodes (1993) was the finding that inclusion of lorazepam, an anxiolytic medication, into an antiemetic treatment for the prevention of chemotherapy-induced nausea/emesis, reduced levels of post-therapy tiredness. It points to anxiety as a possible cause in the development of tiredness and fatigue.

If anxiety is a cause of the development of tiredness, information, education and counseling might be seen as important nursing interventions in preventing tiredness in cancer patients. Self-control through the power of knowledge might prevent feelings of anxiety. It has been proposed that anxiety is alleviated by reducing the extent of the "unknown" by means of information, education and counseling (Glaus and Grahn 1995).

A study by Kaasa and colleagues (1991) has shown that tiredness can disappear with the disappearance of disease at the end of treatment, illustrating that after successful completion of treatment, fatigue does not persist. As a follow-up study of 146 former patients with testicular cancer who were successfully treated with surgery, radiotherapy and chemotherapy, it found that they were not only more satisfied with life but also felt significantly less exhausted after working; they felt even stronger and fitter than an age-matched control group. This finding suggests an improvement of quality of life satisfaction after successful recovery from a potentially mortal disease, which goes along with an improvement in energy resources, however these resources might be defined. The finding also supports the hypothesis that tiredness correlates with type and stage of cancer, indicating that successfully overcoming the disease also means overcoming cancer-related tiredness, whether this tiredness be caused by physical, biochemical or psychological sources.

Conclusions

There is still no universally accepted definition of fatigue. Hypotheses have been developed for the possible underlying mechanisms, involving physiological, neurological and psychological processes in both health and disease. Fatigue can be seen as a protective regulator designed to maintain health and to prevent breakdown. Age and gender, activity and psychological reactions have been discussed as factors that might influence vulnerability to fatigue in both healthy and sick persons. In disease, fatigue becomes a symptom of the impaired body system and of the impact of chronic illness on human life. Whereas it is not yet known for sure whether the chronic fatigue syndrome is best classified as a psychological or a physical diagnosis, there is growing evidence to suggest that depression and anxiety are both factors that may lead to fatigue and that fatigue might lead to depression. In cancer patients, it is evident that physical, biochemical and psychological processes are interwoven. The primary impact of cancer tissue on the organ system of the human body, in addition to secondary causes induced by the tumor itself, such as cytokines, changes in the energy transforming process, and paraneoplastic syndromes, have been proposed as fatigue-inducing factors. The causes of fatigue resulting from cancer therapy, such as surgery, chemotherapy, radiotherapy, and biotherapy, represent a different concept than that of fatigue induced by the tumor itself, even though the delineation between causes seems difficult.

A high prevalence of fatigue in cancer patients is evident from recent publications, but the usefulness of this is unfortunately much hampered by problems in definition and by the variety of methods used in its measurement, which make it difficult to compare the results. Future research needs to address the definition of fatigue/tiredness. What is the experience of tiredness in cancer patients in comparison with tiredness as experienced by healthy individuals? Is there a continuum of fatigue/tiredness in cancer patients that is useful and valid for its measurement? Such knowledge about cancer-specific fatigue/tiredness will serve as a scientific basis against which to identify the validity of the content of a measurement instrument for cancer-specific tiredness. Valid and reliable measurement will eventually make it possible to search for correlations of fatigue levels with possible causes, and eventually to measure the effect of treatment strategies.

References

Adams F, Queseda J (1984) Neuropsychiatric manifestations of human leukocyte interferon therapy in patients with cancer. J Am Med Assoc 252:938–941

Akert K, Koella W (1952) Sleep produced by electrical stimulation of the thalamus. Am J Physiol 168:259–267

Appels A, Mulder P (1988) Excess fatigue as a precursor of myocardial infarction. Eur Heart J 9:758–764

Bafitis H, Sargent F (1977) Human physiological adaptability through the life sequence. Gerontology 324:402–410

Bartley S (1947) Fatigue and impairment in men. McGraw Hill, New York

Bartley SH (1967) The human organism as a person. Chilton, Philadelphia

Behan P, Behan W (1985) The post-viral fatigue syndrome: an analysis of the findings in 50 cases. J Infect Dis 10:211–222

Berrios G (1990) Feelings of fatigue and psychopathology: a conceptual history. Comp Psychiatry 31 (2):140–151

Beutler B, Cerami A (1987) Cachectin: more than a tumor necrosis factor. N Engl J Med 316 379–385

Blesch K, Paice J (1991) Correlates of fatigue in people with breast or lung cancer. Oncol Nurs Forum 18 (1):81–87

Bloom J, Gorsky R (1990) Physical performance at work and at leisure: validation of a measure of biological energy in survivors of Hodgkin's disease. J Psychosoc Oncol 8 (1):49–63

Bodnar R, Pasternak G (1989) Mediation of anorexia by human recombinant tumour necrosis factor through a peripheral action in the rat. Cancer Res 49:6280–6284

Bruera E (1988) Asthenia in patients with advanced cancer. J Pain Sympt Manag 3 (1):9–13

Bruera E, Brenneis C (1988) Muscle electrophysiology in patients with advanced breast cancer. J Natl Cancer Inst 80:282–285

Bruera E, Brenneis C (1989) Association between asthenia and nutritional status lean body mass anemia psychological status and tumor mass in patients with advanced breast cancer. J Pain Sympt Manag 4 (2):59–63

Butow P, Coates A (1991) On the receiving end IV: validation of quality of life indicators. Ann Oncol 2:297–603

Cardenas D, Kutner N (1982) The problem of fatigue in dialysis patients. Nephron 30:336–340

Chen M (1986) The epidemiology of self-perceived fatigue among adults. Prev Med 15:74–81

Cowles E (1893) The mental symptoms of fatigue. NY Med J 1:345–352

Christensen T, Hjortso N (1986) Fatigue and anxiety in surgical patients. Acta Psychiatr Scand 73:76–79

Crosby L (1991) Factors which contribute to fatigue associated with rheumatoid arthritis. J Adv Nurs 16:974–981

Davis C (1984) Interferon-induced fatigue (abstract no 72). Oncol Nurs Forum 11 [Suppl]

David A, Pelosi E (1990) Tired weak or in need of rest: fatigue among general practice attenders. Br Med J 301:1199–1202

Denz H, Orth B (1993) Weight loss in patients with haematological neoplasias is associated with immune system stimulation. Clin Invest 71:37–41

De Wys D, Begg C (1980) Prognostic effect of weight loss prior to chemotherapy in cancer patients. Am J Med 69:491–497
Dill DB (1967) The Harvard fatigue laboratory: its development contributions and demise. Circ Res 20 [Suppl 1]:161–170
Dubos R (1959) The mirage of health. Wiley, Chichester
Duden (1985) Wörterbuch medizinischer Fachausdrücke. Thieme, Stuttgart
Eichel C (1986) Stress and coping in patients on CAPD compared to hemodialysis patients. ANNA J 131:9–13
Engel G, Schmale A (1972) Conservation-withdrawal: a primary regulatory process for organismic homeostasis physiology emotion and psychosomatic illness. Elsevier Exerpta Medica, Amsterdam, pp 57–85 (Ciba Foundation Symposium, vol 8)
Faithfull S (1991) Patients' experience following cranial radiotherapy: a study of the somnolence syndrome. J Adv Nurs 16:939–946
Fawzy F, Cousin N (1990) A structured psychiatry intervention for cancer patients. Arch Gen Psychiatry 47:720–725
Freel M, Hart L (1977) Study of fatigue phenomena of multiple sclerosis patients (USDHEW Grant no 5R02-NU-00534–02). University of Iowa Division of Nursing, Iowa City
Gibson H, Edwards R (1989) Muscular exercise and fatigue. Sports Med 2:121
Glaus A (1993) Assessment of fatigue in cancer- and non-cancer patients and in healthy individuals. Supp Care Cancer 1:305–315
Glaus A, Grahn G (1995) Information education and counselling: essentials of supportive cancer care. In: Klastersky J, Schimpf S, Senn HJ, et al (eds) Handbook of supportive care in cancer. Dekker, New York, pp 437–458
Grandjean E (1961) Die zentrale Ermüdung. In: Lehmann G (ed) Handbuch der gesamten Arbeitsmedizin. Urban and Schwarzenberg, Berlin, pp 442–470
Grandjean E (1968) Fatigue: its physiological and psychological significance. Ergonomics 11:427–436
Greenberg D (1990) Neurasthenia in the 1980's: chronic mononucleosis chronic fatigue syndrome and anxiety and depressive disorders. Psychosomatics 31 (2):129–137
Haeuber D (1989) Recent advances in the management of biotherapy-related side effects: flu-like syndrome. Oncol Nurs Forum 16 [Suppl 6]:35–41
Hart L, Freel M (1982) Fatigue. In: Norris C (ed) Concept clarification in nursing. Aspen, Rockville, pp 251–261
Haylock P, Hart L (1979) Fatigue in patients receiving localized radiation. Cancer Nurs 2:461–467
Hess W (1948) Die funktionelle Organisation des vegetativen Nervensystems. Schwabe, Basel
Holmes S (1991) Preliminary investigation of symptom distress in two cancer patient populations: evaluation of a measurement instrument. J Adv Nurs 16:439–446
Ioteyko J (1920) La fatigue. Flammarion, Paris
Irvine D, Vincent L (1991) A critical appraisal of the research literature investigating fatigue in the individual with cancer. Cancer Nurs 144:188–199
Irvine D, Vincent L (1994) The prevalence and correlates of fatigue in patients receiving treatment with chemotherapy and radiotherapy: a comparison with the fatigue experienced by healthy individuals. Cancer Nurs 17 (5):367–378
Jamar S (1982) Fatigue in women receiving chemotherapy for ovarian cancer. In: Funk S, Tornquist E (eds) Key aspects of comfort. Springer, Berlin Heidelberg New York
Kaasa S, Aass N, Mastekaasa A, Lund E, Fossa SD (1991) Psychological well-being in testicular cancer patients. Eur J Cancer 27:1091–1095
Keller U (1993) Pathophysiology of cancer cachexia. Supp Care Cancer 1:290–294
Kensies F (1898) Arbeitshygiene der Schule auf Grund von Ermüdungsmessen. Reuther and Reichard, Berlin
King K, Nail L (1985) Patients descriptions of the experience of receiving radiation therapy. Oncol Nurs Forum 12:55–61
Knoff M (1986) Physical and psychological distress associated with adjuvant chemotherapy in women with breast cancer. J Clin Oncol 4 (5):678–684

Kraepelin E (1898) Zur Überbürdungsfrage. Fischer, Jena
Kristoffersson A, Boström A (1992) Muscle strength is improved after parathyroidectomy in patients with primary hyperparathyroidism. Br J Surg 79:1165–1168
Kronecker H (1871) Über die Ermüdung und Erholung der quergestreiften Muskeln. Ber Verh Sachs Gesell Wiss Lpg 5:710–736
Krupp L, Alvarez L (1988) Fatigue in multiple sclerosis. Arch Neurol 45:435–437
Lloyd A, Wakefield D (1988) What is myalgic encephalomyelitis? Lancet 6 (4):1286–1287
Love R, Leventhal H (1989) Side effects and emotional distress during cancer chemotherapy. Cancer 63:604–612
McCorkle R, Quint-Benoliel J (1983) Symptom distress current concerns and mood disturbance after diagnosis of life-threatening disease. Soc Sci Med 17 (7):431–438
MacDougall R (1899) Fatigue. Psychol Rev 6:203–208
McNair D, Lorr M (1971) EITS manual for the Profile of Mood States. Educational and Industrial Testing Service, San Diego
Meyerowitz B, Watkins I (1983) Quality of life for breast cancer patients receiving adjuvant chemotherapy. Am J Nurs 83 (2):232–235
Montgomery G (1983) Uncommon tiredness among college undergraduates. J Consult Clin Psychol 51:517–525
Mooney K, Ferrel B, Nail L, et al (1991) Oncology Nursing Society research priorities survey. Oncol Nurs Forum 18 (8):1381–1388
Morant R (1991) Asthenia in cancer patients – a double-edged inflammatory response against the tumor? J Pall Care 7 (3):22–24
Morris M (1982) Tiredness and fatigue. In: Norris C (ed) Concept clarification in nursing. Aspen, Rockville, pp 263–275
Mosso A (1903) La fatigue: intellectuel et physique. Alcan, Paris
Muscio B (1921) Is a fatigue test possible? Br J Psychol 12:31–46
Nail L, Winningham M (1993) Fatigue. In: Groenwald S, Frogge M (eds) Cancer nursing: principles and practice, 3rd edn. Jones and Bartlett, Boston, pp 608–619
Naylor M, Malik S (1990) In situ detection of tumour necrosis factor in human ovarian cancer specimen. Eur J Cancer 26:1027–1030
Nelson J, Charney D (1981) The symptoms of major depressive illness. Am J Psychiatry 138:1–13
Nerenz DR, Leventhal H (1982) Factors contributing to emotional distress during cancer chemotherapy. Cancer 50 (5):1020–1027
Nixon P (1976) The human function curve. Practitioner 217:765–770
ONS News (1996) 11,1: fire, professional education course held, p 1
Pickard-Holley S (1991) Fatigue in cancer patients. Cancer Nurs 14:13–19
Piper B (1993) Fatigue. In: Carrieri V Lindsey A (eds) Pathophysiological phenomena in nursing. Saunders, Philadelphia
Piper B, Lindsey A (1989) Development of an instrument to measure the subjective dimension of fatigue. In: Funk S, Tournquist E (ed) Key aspects of comfort. Springer, Berlin Heidelberg New York, pp 199–280
Piper B, Rieger L (1989) Recent advances in the management of biotherapy-related side effects: fatigue. Oncol Nurs Forum 16 [Suppl 6]:27–32
Piper B, Lindsey A, Dodd M, et al (1987) Fatigue mechanisms in cancer patients: developing nursing theory. Oncol Nurs Forum 14 (6):17–23
Poffenberger A (1928) The effect of continuous work upon output and feelings. J Appl Psychol 12 (5):450–467
Poteliakhoff A (1981) Adrenocortical activity and some clinical findings in acute and chronic fatigue. J Psychosom Res 25 (2):91–95
Reuter P, Reuter C (1995) Thieme leximed: medical dictionary. Thieme, Stuttgart
Rhodes V, Watson P (1988) Patients' descriptions of the influence of tiredness and weakness on self-care abilities. Cancer Nurs 11 (3):186–194
Richardson A (1996) Patterns of fatigue in patients receiving chemotherapy. Eur J Cancer Care [Suppl]
Senn HJ, Drings P (1992) Checkliste Onkologie. Thieme, Stuttgart

Siegl G (1994) Das chronische Erschöpfungssyndrom. IKMI Info Bulletin des Institutes für Klinische Mikrobiologie und Immunologie St. Gallen 12:1–3
Simms S, Rhodes V (1993) Comparison of prochlorperazine and lorazepam antiemetic regimens in the control of postchemotherapy symptoms. Nurs Res 42:234–239
Srivastava R (1989) Fatigue in end stage renal disease patients. In: Funk S, Tornquist E (eds) Key aspects of comfort. Springer, Berlin Heidelberg New York, pp 217–233
Stedman's medical dictionary (1973) 22nd edn. Williams and Wilkins, Baltimore
Stetz K, Haberman M, Holcombe J, et al (1994) Oncology Nursing Society research priority survey. Oncol Nurs Forum 22 (5):785–789
Stiefel F, Morant R (1992) Asthenie bei Tumorkranken. Dtsch Med Wochenschr 117:107–111
St Pierre B, Kaspar C (1992) Fatigue mechanisms in patients with cancer: effects of tumour necrosis factor and exercise on skeletal muscle. Oncol Nurs Forum 19:419–425
Theologides A (1982) Asthenia in cancer. Am J Med 73:1–3
Theologides A (1986) Anorexins asthenins and cachectins in cancer. Am J Med 81:296–298
Waterman G (1919) The treatment of fatigue states. J Abnorm Psychol 4:128–139
Weisman A (1979) Coping with cancer. McGraw Hill, New York
Wells F (1908) A neglected measure of fatigue. Am J Psychol 19:345–358
Winningham N, Nail L (1994) Fatigue and the cancer experience: the state of the knowledge. Oncol Nurs Forum 21 (1):23–36
World Health Organization (1990) Cancer pain relief and palliative care. WHO, Geneva (Technical report series 804)
Yoshitake H (1971) Relations between the symptoms and feelings of fatigue. Ergonomics 14 (1):175–186

A Qualitative Study to Explore the Concept of Fatigue/Tiredness in Cancer Patients and in Healthy Individuals*

Introduction

Theories help to summarize existing knowledge into coherent systems and explain the nature of relationships among variables (Polit and Hungler 1993). The overall purpose of theory is to make scientific findings meaningful and generalizable (Chalmers 1982). Fatigue theorists have defined fatigue in healthy persons as a nonspecific state indicative of a decreased level of vitality, which has the protective function of forcing the body to avoid further stress. It is said to allow recovery to take place, with exhaustion being the end of the fatigue continuum, forcing the body to stop functioning (Grandjean 1970). In patients with cancer, fatigue is known to be one of the major distressing symptoms (World Health Organisation 1990). Some theoretical frameworks are available to conceptualize fatigue in cancer patients (Piper 1993; Astair 1987; Cimprich 1992; Winningham et al. 1994; Irvine 1994) and have advanced fatigue research considerably. Further theoretical and empirical work is still needed to define and test causal relationships.

A major problem is the lack of a common scientific language to designate the problem of fatigue in cancer patients. There is also no clear definition of the continuum of tiredness or fatigue. For example, what is a deviation from "normal" tiredness? What is "acceptable" fatigue in specific circumstances? If tiredness is a phenomenon in healthy as well as in diseased persons, is there a difference in its perception? Does tiredness precede fatigue? It could be argued that when tiredness is perceived as an unusual, continuing distress, it is fatigue rather than tiredness. In the German language, tiredness (*Müdigkeit*) is not the same as fatigue (*Ermüdung*). The German translation of fatigue is thus comparable to "fatiguability" (*Ermüdbarkeit*) or to getting tired, suggesting that it is the consequence of unrelieved tiredness or "fatiguability," which leads to exhaustion (*Erschöpfung*) (Weis 1990). It could then be said that it is the illness feeling of unusual tiredness that represents "problematic or distressing tiredness" in diseased persons, such as cancer patients. The continuum could range from "no unusual tiredness" (*keine ungewöhnliche Müdigkeit*), through easy tiring (*leichte Ermüdbarkeit*), to extreme, unusual tiredness (*extreme, unübliche Müdigkeit*), to exhaustion (*Erschöpfung*). This

* This chapter was coauthored by Rosemary Crow and Hammond Sean.

definition is in accordance with Piper's statement that "in contrast to tiredness, subjective fatigue is perceived as unusual, abnormal or excessive whole-body tiredness, disproportionate to or unrelated to activity or exertion" (Piper 1993). As fatigue is a foreign word in the German language, in this research its operational term is simply "extreme tiredness."

Concepts thus play an important part in the development of knowledge. The concept of fatigue/tiredness is still unclear as it represents a variety of unrelated phenomena (Funk in Piper and Lindsey 1989). Its measurement and treatment therefore require a definition of these phenomena. The question still needing an answer is: "What is the fatigue/tiredness that is experienced by cancer patients?"

Aims

The aim of this study was to explore the concept of fatigue/tiredness from the native's perspective in order to:
- Learn about the lived experience of tiredness/fatigue in cancer patients
- Compare cancer patients' experience with that of healthy individuals
- Generate theoretical knowledge concerning cancer-specific tiredness/fatigue

Methods

Research Approach and Design

In order to learn from the individuals' experience of tiredness, a qualitative method was used. Qualitative methods are particularly useful when describing a phenomenon from the perspective of the person concerned, that is, the perspective of the problem from the "native's point of view" (Harris 1968). Understanding tiredness is difficult, because its experience is subjective, multidimensional and difficult to measure quantitatively. This becomes especially true in view of the vulnerability of cancer patients, whose disease may not only entail physical suffering but represents a life crisis. Symptoms such as tiredness might therefore be perceived and expressed in many different ways. Qualitative methods allow understanding, "verstehen," by means of an individual's empathy, intuition or imagination, and therefore go beyond knowledge obtained by means of observation or calculation (Melia 1992). Such an approach seems mandatory in any attempt to understand a complex, subjective experience such as tiredness/fatigue.

Phenomenology or Grounded Theory?

Phenomenology is rooted in the philosophical tradition. It is a descriptive approach to research and has the objective of identifying the essence of behavior, based on meditative thought. Its purpose is to promote an understanding of human beings wherever they may be found (Omery 1983) and hence to generate theories, models or a general explanation (Field and Morse 1994). Although this approach might have seemed appropriate, the results would not have provided descriptions of the experience of the phenomenon under study.

Grounded theory represents a methodology designed to achieve an accurate description. The central idea of this approach is that theory is generated from and grounded in data by a process of induction, thus assuming the existence of a process. Glaser and Strauss (1967) argue that the collected data serve to generate rather than to prove a hypothesis. Theory generation rather than verification is thus the ultimate aim of the grounded approach. As it was also the intention to discover dominant (exploratory) processes rather than merely describe observations, an intention attributed to grounded theory, this theory was the preferred method. A further reason for choosing grounded theory was that fatigue and tiredness in cancer patients is not yet thoroughly understood.

It is apparent from the literature that selected aspects of both methodologies are confused and, in particular, susceptible to the "blurring trend" observed by Morse (1989). This means that elements can be interchanged. Clarke (1995) suggests that the technique of grounded theory is not wholly incompatible with the Popperian method, in that a deductive element is inherent in the underlying theory. Chenitz (1994) agrees, saying that it is based upon the judicious use of induction, deduction and intuition. Phenomenology and grounded theory research approaches are based on different assumptions and therefore differ in purpose and methodological descriptions (Baker et al. 1992). The reluctance to apply a methodology based on a strict grounded theory approach may reflect the fact that Glaser and Strauss (1967) did not clearly describe the analytical capacity of their conception.

This study used an exploratory approach because little is yet known about the experience of tiredness from the perspective of the persons concerned. Questions such as "what is it" or "what does it feel like" seemed appropriate to an attempt at further understanding of the concept. Hypothesis and theories were not preconceived but were allowed to emerge from the data while data collection was in progress and after data analysis had commenced (Field and Morse 1994). An analysis of the literature, especially that concerning the fatigue measurement tools, suggested there was a lack of unbiased research. Findings from the data were then compared with available knowledge.

Setting, Selection and Sample

The study took place within the oncology department of a teaching hospital in Switzerland. Cancer patients were selected weekly on ward rounds according to their availability. The selection criteria were: oral consent to the conduct of an interview with the nurse researcher, possession of the necessary cognitive ability to report their experience and ability to speak the German language. In accordance with qualitative strategies, no variables were controlled when selecting interviewees apart from (a) the exclusion of patients with brain tumors, as they might have been affected cognitively and (b) gender, as it might have an influence on the experience of tiredness (Glaus 1993). Qualitative appropriateness requires purposeful sampling, which was thus adopted, as participants were selected according to the needs of the study (Morse 1991).

The data collection period in the group of cancer patients was August and September 1994. Data saturation was achieved with interview data collected from 20 cancer patients. Data saturation refers to the sense of closure that the researcher experiences when data collection ceases to yield any new information (Polit and Hungler 1993). It confirmed Glaser's (1978) view that to obtain a full account of the phenomena under study 20–50 interviews are necessary to elicit major, repetitive themes relating to the topic.

The interviews with healthy individuals followed in November 1994 to January 1995. The selection of the healthy individuals was determined by availability of willing persons in the working and personal environment of the nurse researcher, and the same criteria applied: oral consent to the conduct of an interview and ability to speak and understand the German language. Purposeful sampling was again the selection of choice, but was subject to a sampling frame of age and gender variables to make sure that the healthy group was similar in age and gender to the patient group. The healthy individuals were included only if they did not suffer from chronic disease, in order to ensure the difference between cancer patients and healthy persons. To ensure a comparable number of interviews in this group, data collection was continued until 20 interviews had been conducted; data saturation have been well achieved at that stage.

The study was approved by the ethical committee of the hospital and permission was obtained from the head of department. Patients and healthy persons gave oral consent and were assured of confidentiality. A numbered participant list was kept separately from other information material. Identification of interviewees was not allowed either on the tape or on the transcript.

Instruments and Procedures

The Interview Method

The interview method, a predominant mode of data collection in qualitative research, was used to collect information. As the aim of the study was to uncover the feelings, experiences and words of "the real fatigue-world," interviewees were given the opportunity to speak spontaneously about their experience. Qualitative studies typically employ unstructured or semistructured interviews to avoid reflecting preconceived ideas about content and flow and can be undertaken with little or no organization (Morse 1991). For the purpose of this study and in accordance with the grounded theory approach, the interviews were unstructured. Previous knowledge and experience were therefore subordinated as "hidden agenda" (Oppenheim 1992) to the process of discovering each informant's perspectives on tiredness. The later interviews in the study became more structured as the preliminary findings enabled questioning to become more focused. Topics for the questions were derived from the initial process of conceptualization, with further ones added during the course of the interviews.

Even though the interviews themselves were unstructured, three leading questions on the "hidden agenda" were asked if subjects did not mention the topics spontaneously. The topics concerned: the occurrence of weakness, the occurrence of malaise, and the linguistic description of tiredness. This deductive part of the study was carried out to compare the occurrence of these concepts with findings in the existing literature (Kobashi et al. 1985).

All interviews were conducted by the same nurse researcher on a one-time basis and scheduled for a convenient time. Most patient interviews took place in the patient's room, or if there was a need for privacy or to prevent interruption, in the researcher's office. They varied in length from 30 to 50 min. Open questions such as "what is it?" or "what does it feel like?" challenged the informants to talk about their own experience. Interviewing cancer patients about tiredness put an emotional strain on many of them, as it concerned feelings of loss and coping with progressive disease. This was acknowledged by the researcher by giving patients time for sobbing, slowly going back to discussion of more superficial topics. Maintenance of rapport and trust was considered to be important, in order to keep the patients talking while at the same time maintaining their psychological well-being.

The interviews with healthy persons were emotionally less strenuous, even though they often became very personal. Many admitted that they would not normally tell people that they felt tired.

All interviews were tape-recorded with the subjects' permission. They showed no signs of "stage fright" once the interview had started. Field notes were made to record special events. The whole text was transcribed by the nurse researcher to allow her to become familiar with the data.

Collection of Biomedical Information; the Karnofsky Index

Data concerning gender, age, type and stage of disease and current treatment of the cancer patient group were collected from the medical records to assess comparability between individuals. Performance status was assessed by the nurse investigator with the aid of the Karnofsky Index Scale. This numerical scale from 0 to 100 represents the patient's ability to perform normal activity and to do active work and his or her need for assistance; it has been widely tested and used in clinical decision making (Schag et al. 1984). The index was used to assess the impact of the disease on the individuals' activity and their need for assistance.

Data Analysis

The analytical process in grounded theory does not differ greatly from the processes used in other qualitative approaches. Researchers organize the data, analyze the content and search for integrative themes and patterns (Polit and Hungler 1993). The main difference lies in the fact that in the grounded approach, data collection and analysis occur concurrently based on the constant comparative method, which is seen as generating theory from data or the discovery of grounded theory (Glaser and Strauss 1967). This is in contrast with the generation of a conceptual framework from previous studies.

The purpose of this study was to generate constructs that would describe or explain the phenomenon of fatigue/tiredness. Analysis started soon after the first interviews. The researcher read the transcripts line by line, looking for significant incidents or phenomena. Persistent words, phrases, themes or concepts were recognized and identified for later retrieval with a highlighter pen. Themes were identified and numbers assigned to them in the text to identify appropriate content (Miles and Hubermann 1984). The significant passages, marked with the interview number and the line, were then extracted and filed separately under emerging codes and categories. To ensure reliability, a second researcher separately judged the assignment of codes to the significant passages.

The identified themes of the analyzed interviews were then compared with the data subsequently collected. As more information became available, themes had to be partially revised, the emerging concepts then sharpening the focus of the study. Categories were generated by clustering themes that seemed to fit together. It soon became apparent that the expression of tiredness could be grouped at physical, cognitive and affective levels.

To organize the data, the emerging themes were registered in a binary matrix. This allowed the recognition of specific fatigue patterns per person and of the frequencies with which each theme occurred.

Descriptive statistics were used to describe and present data.

Reliability and Validity

Qualitative research methodologies offer valuable approaches to the understanding of human experience. Grounded theory analysis used in this study was consistent with this research approach, providing narrative as opposed to statistical material. The important question concerning validity is thus the trustworthiness of the data. A procedure to evaluate the quality of data in qualitative research is the use of four criteria to establish its trustworthiness: credibility, transferability, dependability and confirmability (Lincoln and Guba 1985). The evaluation of these criteria will be discussed later.

Interrater reliability was established for the coding frame by identification of codes related to significant passages from the interview texts by a second

Table 1. Sample characteristics

Characteristics	Cancer patients ($n=20$)	Healthy individuals ($n=20$)
Gender		
Female	45%	50%
Male	55%	50%
Age		
Mean	66	56
Range	42–81	29–70
Disease state[a]		
Progressive	75%	
Stable	25%	
Tumor therapy		
Yes	85%	
No	15%	
Karnofsky Index		
>70	40%	
<70	60%	

[a] Fourteen different types of cancer.

researcher. The percentage of agreement between the two researchers was 95% in the group with healthy persons and 93% in cancer patients.

Results

Sample Characteristics

The two samples consisted of 20 diseased and 20 healthy individuals. The mean age (66 years) was higher in the patient group than in the group of healthy individuals (56 years). There was an equal distribution between males and females in both samples. Seventy-five percent of patients suffered from active, progressive disease, and 85% were undergoing tumor therapy, mainly chemotherapy. Fourteen different types of malignant tumors were registered. The Karnofsky Index revealed a severe impact of disease in 60% of these patients. In all the healthy individuals the Karnofsky Index was 100% (Table 1).

Cancer Patients

Emerging Concepts of Fatigue/Tiredness

The number of themes addressed in the 20 interviews with cancer patients was 220 (multiple nominations possible), from which the 16 themes were developed. After the analysis of the first interviews, categories started to emerge as it became apparent that sensations of fatigue/tiredness were expressed as either physical, affective or cognitive experiences. This was based on differences between the expressions of tiredness in physical functioning and physical sensations, those of emotional feelings, and those that indicated problems in thinking. Even though the distribution across the three categories was different for individual patients, the distinction between them remained robust to the end of data collection.

Occurrence, Frequency and Distribution of Identified Themes

Table 2 shows the 16 themes that were identified and how they were distributed across the three main categories. Figure 1 shows the occurrence and frequency of the themes from each in cancer patients. Physical sensations were described most frequently (59%) followed by affective sensations (29%) with cognitive sensations being the least frequent (12%) (Fig. 2). Theme 16, malaise, was considered to be a separate concept as it was difficult to assign to any of the other categories.

Table 2. Themes and categories of tiredness identified in cancer patients ($n=20$)

Physical sensations of tiredness (59% of all themes)	
1	Decreased physical performance (18/20)
2	Weakness/no strength (17/20)
3	Unusual need for sleep (more than before illness) (6/20)
4	Unusually tired (more than before illness), feeling worn-out (18/20)
5	Unusual need for rest (more than before illness) (15/20)
Affective sensations of tiredness (29% of all themes)	
6	Decreased motivation (7/20)
7	Need to force oneself to overcome inactivity (5/20)
8	No energy (5/20)
9	Sadness (11/20)
10	Anxiety (4/20)
11	No fighting spirit (4/20)
Cognitive sensations of tiredness (12% of all themes)	
12	Lack of concentration (4/20)
13	Problems in thinking (4/20)
14	Tired in the head (4/20)
15	Sleeping problems at night (3/20)
16	Malaise (2/20)

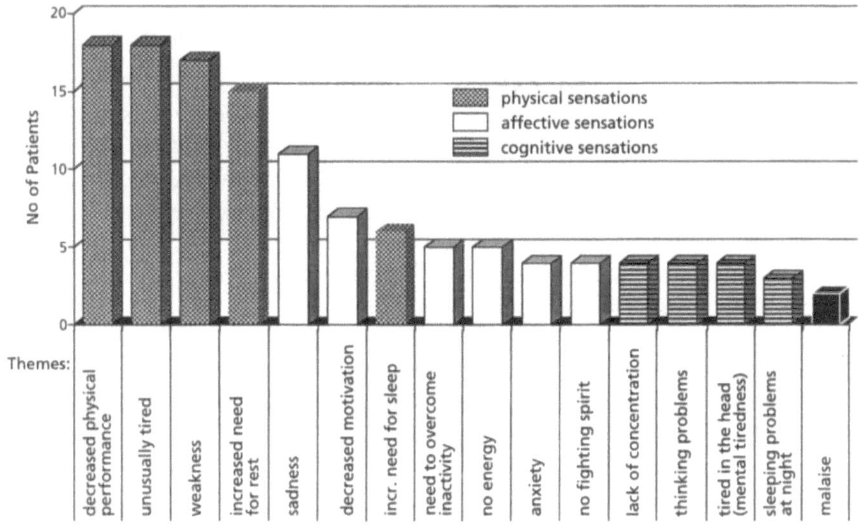

Fig. 1. Occurrence and frequency of themes in cancer patients ($n=20$)

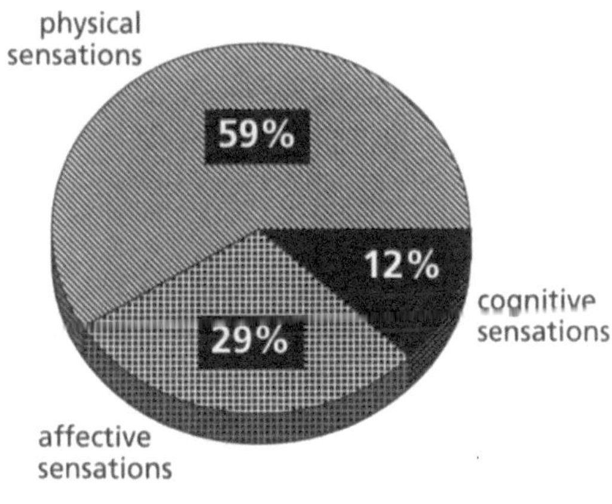

Fig. 2. Fatigue: percentages of physical, affective, and cognitive sensations in cancer patients ($n=20$)

Descriptions of Experiences Expressed

Decreased physical performance (theme 1) and feeling unusually tired and worn out were the most prominent sensations reported. Such feelings were often associated with an inability to walk as far as before or with an inability to do physical activities as before. Typical descriptions (English translations of the German responses) for decreased physical performance included:

"When I walked up the stairs, I thought I wouldn't make it any more."

"I just could not walk as far as I used to."

"Walking to the bathroom makes me feel extremely tired."

"The trip I have planned is a quarter as strenuous as I am used to."

"I wonder how I did all the work last year at Christmas."
"It was only 7 minutes' walk from my flat, and I thought if only I were there already!"

Feeling unusually tired (theme 4) was categorized as a physical sensation, as patients indicated that this form of tiredness described a lack of strength to carry on as usual and was experienced as a bodily sensation. It was expressed mostly by the simple word "tired," in combination with an amplifying adverb. The following expressions were typical:
"I feel unusually tired," "madly tired," "finished."
"It is difficult to explain, simply tired."
"More and more tired," "dead tired," "so tired," "very tired," "terribly tired."
"I have been tired in the past, but never so much as now."
"Constantly tired," "omnipresent tiredness," "heavily tired."
"My whole body is shattered," "worn out," "tired in every limb."
"Tired from morning to night."

Weakness (theme 2) was equated with no strength and was the third most frequently mentioned concept. The overwhelming impact of it as an experience is described by the following quotes:
"Tiredness feels similar to weakness," "it feels weak, weak..."
"I had no strength any more," "I feel much weaker than before."
"I do not regain strength, I feel weak," "it's weakness, only weakness..."
"Tiredness comes from weakness," "through tiredness I become weak."

Unusual need for rest (theme 5), the fourth most frequently occurring theme, could mean the need for the persons affected either to stop what they were doing and sit down or otherwise have a break, or to lie down for a rest. Typical quotes were:
"I am always on the lookout for a chance to sit down."
"Then you only want to lie down, to close your eyes and rest, and that wish becomes an addiction."
"I have problems with walking, I need to rest in between."
"Then I just can't any more and I lie down," "I want to lie down, anywhere."
"If I work in the garden, suddenly it feels as though the gasoline ran out and nothing works any more; I then need to lie down and wait until some gasoline runs in again."

Sadness (theme 9) is the most frequently identified affective sensation. Feelings of sadness were expressed by words or nonverbal expressions such as crying. Examples of verbal expressions were:
"Tiredness feels like depression, it makes me feel listless, one has to fight against it."
"Sometimes I feel sad because I cannot do as I used to."
"Fatigue is a physical experience but there is also something psychological; if one thinks of being a candidate for dying, it doesn't cheer you up."
"I am of no use at anything any more."
"I have no interest any more in what is going on in the world."

The remaining themes from the affective category (6, 7, 8, 10, and 11) describe the concepts of loss of motivation, the fight to overcome inactivity, loss of energy, anxiety and a sense of fighting spirit.

Cognitive sensations included lack of concentration, problems in thinking, "tiredness in the head" (i.e., a tired mind) (themes 12 and 13). They appeared less prominent than all other categories even though their impact seemed to be severe. Some quotes illustrate the impact:

"You're tired in your head, you like closing your eyes."
"I cannot go on thinking, I am too tired."
"You forget things, have difficulty concentrating."
"I can't keep my thoughts in order properly "
"Your brain doesn't function."

Sleeping problems at night (theme 15) were mentioned by three patients, making integration into a category difficult. Malaise (theme 16) was not identified spontaneously by cancer patients; two of them recognized it when asked a question about it. A most interesting report came from a young male cancer patient, who explained the experience of tiredness/fatigue in the following words:

"It is in the limbs, but also in the head, you're too listless to read a newspaper or to watch television, it is 'total tiredness.'"

Individual Patterns

Individual patterns of fatigue were documented on a binary matrix. The overall distribution of themes reported varied from person to person. Only the physical sensations appeared consistently throughout all the interviews.

Linguistic Description of Tiredness

A linguistic exploration of how Swiss patients labeled their tiredness is presented in Table 3 (translated from Swiss-German). It reflects the words used by the patients to describe what they perceived as tiredness.

Healthy Individuals

Emerging Concepts of Fatigue/Tiredness

Interviews with the healthy persons were easier to conduct; their length was between 15 and 30 min and they usually did not stir up deep emotional feelings. One hundred and forty-one descriptions were identified from the interviews, fewer than in the group of cancer patients (220). After analysis of the first interviews, the same three categories as in the sample of cancer patients seemed appropriate, even though not all the themes were the same. Criteria used to assign themes to a category were the distinction between physical, cognitive or affective expression.

Table 3. Linguistic analysis: words to describe "feeling tired" (*müde*) identified by 20 cancer patients (translated from Swiss-German)

• I wouldn't know a better word than tired. I usually say: I feel so tired I have to lie down
• Worn out, worn out, it's (even) more than worn out
• No strength, no appetite, depressed mood
• One does not know what is coming: uncertainty causes stress
• It is difficult to explain
• I do not feel well
• To be worn-out, shattered
• Indifference, listlessness
• Yes, it (tired) is the right word. Energy is reduced
• To be dissatisfied, indecisive, changeable, out of balance, aggressive? irritable
• Could not find another, better word than tired, worn out (*schlapp*)
• Lazy, always lazy!
• Cannot find another word than "tired"
• I could hardly keep going any more
• Desire to rest

Occurrence, Frequency and Distribution of Identified Themes

Table 4 shows the 16 themes that were used to code the data and their distribution into three categories. There were seven physical sensations (themes 1–7), four affective sensations (themes 8–11) and four cognitive sensations (themes 12–15). The concepts of malaise (theme 16) and weakness (theme 7) were responses to leading questions in this group if they were not mentioned spontaneously.

Tiredness after a day's work as a rhythmic normality (theme 1) was the most frequently mentioned (in 18 of 20 persons). This was often related to pleasant, relaxing tiredness. Having heavy limbs, legs, and eyelids (theme 5) was ranked second in frequency and occurred as a consequence of work. Sleepiness (theme 14) was reported as something that comes suddenly, and many individuals related it to the evening, when watching television. A typical description was the following:

> "I do not feel tiredness as such, I just suddenly fall asleep (while watching television)."

Tiredness as a pleasant phenomenon, after a special physical exertion (theme 2) was as frequent as was the loss of concentration or attentiveness and forgetting easily (theme 12). Loss of concentration and attentiveness was mostly related to a situation after a working day. The same was the case with the wish to lie down (theme 3). Affective sensations were not mentioned very often apart from the feeling of impatience and irritability (theme 11). Two peo-

Table 4. Themes and categories of tiredness identified in healthy individuals ($n=20$)

Physical sensations of tiredness (55% of all themes)	
1	Tiredness after a day's work, as a rhythmic normality (18/20)
2	Tiredness after physical exercise, as pleasant phenomenon (7/20)
3	The wish to go to bed, to lie down, to rest, silence (6/20)
4	Becoming slower (5/20)
5	Having heavy limbs, legs, eyelids (11/20)
6	Feeling exhausted, worn-out, unable to keep going (2/20)
7	Weakness (asked question) (0/20)
Affective sensations of tiredness (21% of all themes)	
8	Loss of energy, interest (3/20)
9	Feeling depressive (4/20)
10	Wanting to withdraw, to avoid problems (3/20)
11	Feeling impatient, irritable (6/20)
Cognitive sensations of tiredness (24% of all themes)	
12	Loss of concentration, forgetting easily, loss of attentiveness (7/20)
13	Difficulty in finding words, speaking (1/20)
14	Sleepiness (8/20)
15	Thoughts going around in the head (before falling asleep), a wish to "switch off" (5/20)
16	Malaise (when specifically asked about it) (2/20)

ple mentioned malaise (theme 16), identifying it as a problem. None of the healthy subjects felt that they were affected by weakness (theme 7). Figure 3 shows the occurrence and frequency of the themes from each category of the healthy individuals. Of the healthy individuals, 55% identified physical sensations of fatigue/tiredness, 21% identified affective sensations, and 24% indicated cognitive sensations (Fig. 4).

Individual Patterns

Individual patterns were documented again on a binary matrix. No uniform pattern could be recognized, every individual having his/her own experience of fatigue.

Linguistic Description of Tiredness

A linguistic exploration of how healthy individuals labeled their tiredness is presented in Table 5 (translated from Swiss-German). It reflects the words used by the healthy subjects to describe what they perceived as tiredness.

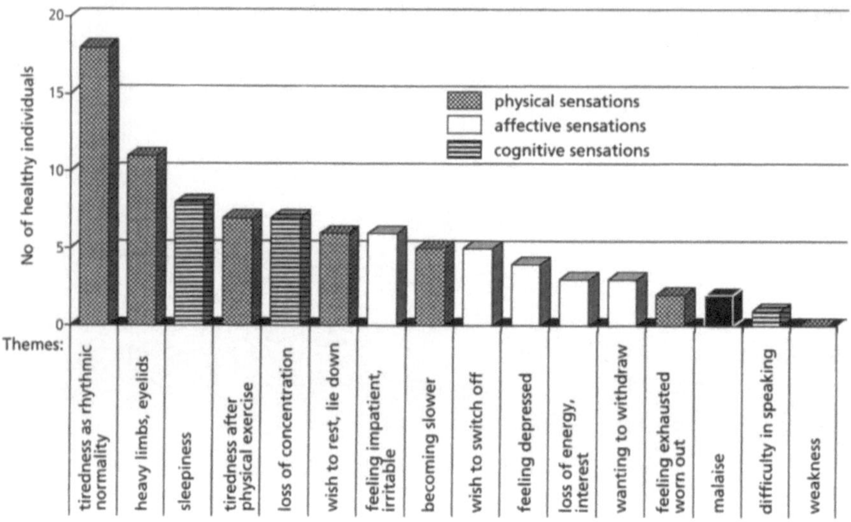

Fig. 3. Occurrence and frequency of themes in healthy persons ($n=20$)

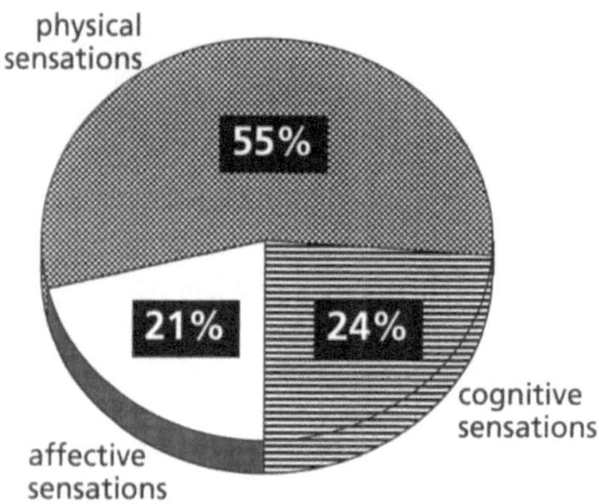

Fig. 4. Fatigue: percentages of physical, affective, and cognitive elements in healthy individuals ($n=20$)

Comparison of the Fatigue Experience of Healthy Individuals and of Cancer Patients

The Themes Identified in Both Subpopulations

Table 6 shows the themes of both groups, ranked according to frequency. It reveals that different physical sensations of tiredness are dominant in both groups. However, whereas healthy people's tiredness is experienced as a circadian rhythm, indicated by limbs heavy from daily activity and by feeling sleepy after work, the cancer patients' experience encompassed decreased physical performance, feeling unusually and extremely tired or weak, and

Table 5. Linguistic analysis: words to describe "feeling tired" (*müde*) identified by 20 healthy individuals (translated from Swiss-German)

• I feel KO (knocked out). I am at zero. Feel the need to go to bed
• I might say: I did not feel well today
• Shattered, ready to go to bed, need silence, to switch off
• I was glad to be able to lie down
• I would not speak about that . . . I would say: I am not very well today
• That depends on who asks the question (in response to: Would you say why?)
• I was lying flat, I also would say tired
• I am at point zero. I've about had it. I want to lie down, to close my eyes and rest
• I need to switch off, to rest, relax, doing nothing more
• I can't go on, do not find the words, can't join in the discussion, feel dazed. There is no productive power
• I was completely finished
• I was shattered, down, exhausted, tired. Tiredness says: it is enough, you must stop
• I am so tired and still cannot sleep, the thoughts turn around in my head
• I was very tired
• I was very tired, it was time to hit the sack
• I am ready to go to bed
• I was lying flat like mad
• I was tired, didn't feel like doing anything
• I have had enough, my capacity is at its limit
• Attentiveness decreases, also the level of being awake
• I was dead tired

needing more rest. These highest ranked themes in both groups characterize the impact of tiredness and illustrate the difference between "healthy tiredness" and tiredness as a form of distress. The affective and cognitive themes appear to be similar for both groups, so that even though tiredness is expressed at physical, affective and cognitive levels in both study samples, the nature of the identified themes reveals a difference between healthy tiredness and tiredness associated with disease.

Weakness and Malaise in the Two Subpopulations

Malaise was either denied by most subjects in both groups or it was unclear; only two persons in each group felt that "*Unwohlsein*," the German version of malaise, was a reality (Fig. 5). Figure 6 shows that weakness was a prominent concept associated with fatigue/tiredness in cancer patients, with 85% stating that it occurred. None of the healthy persons felt weak.

Table 6. Themes of tiredness identified in the two study samples (from open interviews)

Themes of tiredness:			
In healthy individuals[a] ($n=20$)	n	In cancer patients[b] ($n=20$)	n
Tiredness after a working day, rhythmic event	18	Decreased physical performance	18
Heavy limbs, eyelids	11	Unusually tired, more than before illness	18
Sleepiness	8	Weakness, no strength	17
Impaired concentration, loss of attentiveness, forgetting easily	7	Unusual need for rest, more than before illness	15
Tiredness after physical exercise, pleasant	7	Sadness	11
Wishing to go to bed, lie down, rest	6	Decreased motivation	7
Feeling impatient, irritable	6	Unusual need for sleep, more than before illness	6
Becoming slower	5	Need to force oneself to overcome inactivity	5
Thoughts revolving in one's head while trying to fall asleep	5	Anxiety	4
Feeling depressive	4	No energy	5
Loss of energy, interest	3	No fighting spirit	4
Wishing to withdraw	3	Problems with thinking	4
Feeling exhausted, worn-out, unable to keep going	2	Lack of concentration	4
		Tired in the head (mental)	4
Difficulty finding words or speaking	1	Sleeping problems at night	3

[a] Weakness: 12 no, 8 unclear; malaise: 2 yes, 13 no, 5 unclear.
[b] Weakness: 17 yes, 3 no; malaise: 2 yes, 13 no, 5 unclear.

Discussion

What Is It Like to Live Through the Experience of Tiredness/Fatigue?

The value of this qualitative research project lies in the insight it has given into the experience of tiredness as lived by cancer patients and healthy individuals. No existing measurement instrument or conceptual model directed the investigation, as the aim was to learn from the data to make a definition of tiredness/fatigue according to the experience of the study subjects possible. The richness of the data obtained reflects the appropriateness of using this grounded analysis approach, allowing data from the perspective of those concerned to be compared with existing theory.

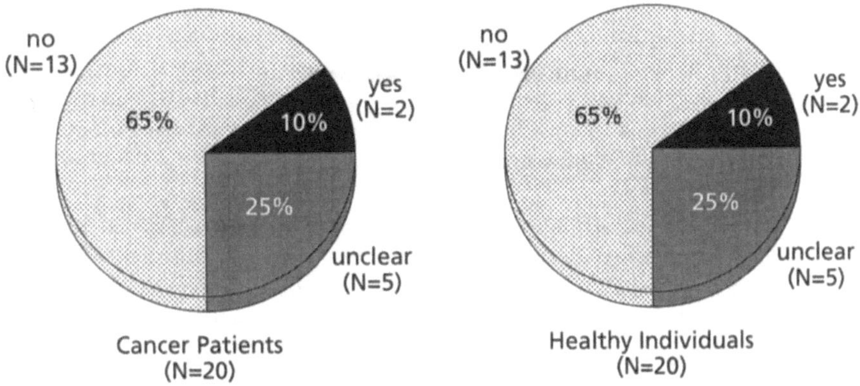

Fig. 5. Occurrence of malaise in cancer patients and healthy individuals (in percent)

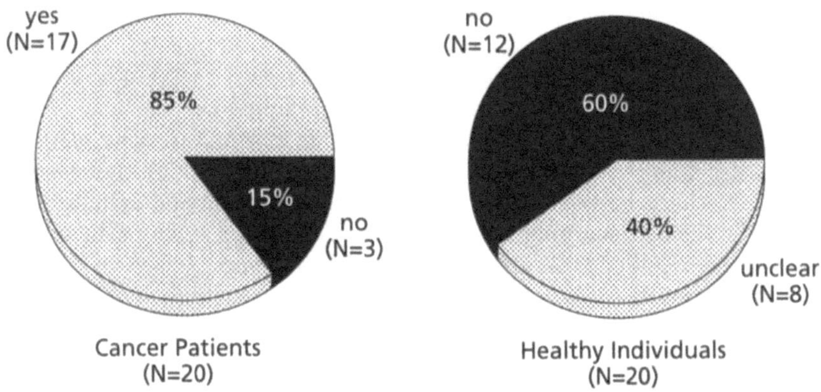

Fig. 6. Occurrence of weakness in cancer patients and healthy individuals (in percent)

Emerging Concepts in Cancer Patients and Their Relation to Existing Theories

The concepts that emerged were different for cancer patients than for the healthy individuals. Most of the cancer patients expressed the four most prominent, distressing concepts of tiredness within a physical frame of reference, such as decreased physical performance, feeling unusually, extremely tired and weak and in unusual need of rest. Decreased physical performance was frequently expressed as an inability to walk as far as before. Patients said they used energy-saving activities, such as swimming or cycling rather than walking, to take exercise or provide mobility albeit with decreased performance, so that they were still able to support well-being. One of the patient's comments, "I wonder how I did all the work I did before," suggests that patients compare their state with the way things were before their illness. Patients described both intensity and duration of the signs as abnormal or unusual. The fact that patients express physical experiences of tiredness as decreased strength looks as though it may be a key dimension that needs to be isolated, as it could be an independent feature of tiredness. Most of the patients in this study suffered from advanced cancer disease and their Karnofsky Index was low. A low Karnofsky Index has been shown by Schag et al. (1984) to correlate significantly with evidence of disease and intensity of reduced energy.

How can decreased strength or reduced energy be defined? What kind of energy is lacking, when decreased physical performance, unusual tiredness, weakness or unusual need for sleep interferes with daily living? The energy analysis model described by Irvine (1995) offers a theoretical explanation. In this model, energy is defined as the capacity to do work on biological, psychological, cognitive and social levels. Humans depend on internal sources (e.g., sleep, rest, motivation, spirituality) and external sources (e.g., food, water, air) for their energy. The availability of energy in the system is determined by the body's physiological processing and its distribution. It is possible, therefore, that pathophysiological changes might disrupt the process of energy transformation. Cancer treatment, symptom-induced distress and mood disturbances are described as energy response modifiers in Irvine's model, representing a constellation of factors unique to cancer that can modify sources of energy, its transformation and its expenditure. The model postulates that cancer cachexia represents a change in the energy transformation processes, characterized by loss of body weight, fatigue and activity intolerance. The themes emerging from the interviews in this study partially fit this framework, with unusual tiredness, activity intolerance such as decreased motivation, the need to force oneself to overcome inactivity, and an unusual need for rest and sleep being attributes associated with a lack of energy.

While the prominent occurrence of weakness could be seen as activity intolerance, it is also possible that further energy response modifiers are responsible for activity intolerance. For example, Morant (1991) considers cytokines, such as asthenins, cachectins, interferons, interleukin-2 and other, unknown, substances produced by the tumor or the immune system (as inflammatory response of the body against the tumor), as possible factors. Irvine's definition can be seen from a physical, psychological or social perspective. Since it could also be argued that not all cancer patients experience weight loss, fatigue or activity intolerance, it is possible that fatigue/tiredness may be related either to the type and/or stage of disease or to individual factors, or to a combination of both the disease and individual factors.

Physical expression of fatigue/tiredness was the most frequent and prominent feature within this study. Whether this finding can be generalized needs to be tested. It could be argued that patients find it easier to talk about physical experiences rather than their psychological experiences, a finding reported by other researchers (Kobashi et al. 1985). Apart from the physical signs of tiredness, some, less prominent psychological concepts emerged (Table 2). Sadness was verbally or nonverbally expressed by 11 of the 20 patients. Whether sadness is an independent concept correlated with tiredness or simply an expression of tiredness cannot yet be answered. It is evident from clinical experience that cancer affects patients not only physically, but also psychologically and socially. Anxiety has also been expressed, and decreased motivation may be psychologically based. The theoretical framework developed by Piper pays attention to the multidimensionality of fatigue by describing the perceptual, physiological, biochemical and behavioral manifestation of fatigue, recognizing the many potential causes and factors that influence it (Piper 1993). The theoretical framework, however, does not specify the relationship between the responses and the aspects which influence them, indicating the complexity of the phenomenon. Our data suggest that the affective expression of fatigue might be strongly interwoven with the physical dimension. This raises a question of whether there is a vicious circle, where sadness leads to tiredness (or vice versa), which then leads to decreased motivation and inactivity (or vice versa), with the inactivity then leading to sadness (or vice versa).

The concepts concerned with problems in thinking, lack of concentration, and a tired mind, all of which emerged in our study, could be interpreted as the cognitive manifestation of tiredness. Patients appeared to suggest that some of these cognitive functions felt as though they were partially out of their control as indicated by the quote from one of the patients: "my brain isn't functioning." Cimprich's theory of attentional fatigue links increased requirements or demands for directed attention with the development of attentional fatigue (Cimprich 1992). She postulates that when demands exceed the available capacity the person affected is at risk of attentional fatigue. This form of fatigue could result in reduced effectiveness in basic cognitive or mental activities, such as acquiring information, planning, problem-solving, and performing tasks of daily living. For cancer patients, the demand for informational, affective and behavioral factors made by the disease and its treatment may increase the need for attention over long periods.

Further support for the cognitive expression of tiredness is given by Gibson and Edwards (1985) in the two types of neurophysiological mechanisms that might be related to tiredness. One of these is a central mechanism (related to the brain, psyche and spinal cord) and the second is a peripheral mechanism (related to peripheral nerves, muscles and other influencing factors related to metabolites, electrolytes and others). It remains unclear, however, whether the central or peripheral mechanisms in cancer patients are caused by the disease itself or the therapeutic interventions, or whether the demands imposed on the individual by the burden of coping with the disease exceed available capacity. Fatigue has also been described as a "dose-limiting factor" of treatment with various biotherapeutic agents regarded as causing mental fatigue and cognitive deficits (Piper and Rieger 1989). Since in our study none of the patients received biotherapeutic treatment, there must be other causes of cognitive dysfunction. For example, as the body itself produces biological response modifiers in order to fight the tumor (Morant 1991), expressions of tiredness could be seen as a sign of tumor activity.

The unusual need for sleep described by our patients fits in with the theoretical model incorporating the reticular activating system proposed by Astair (1987). The reticular activating system (RAS) is located in the reticular formation of the midbrain and medulla and is known to be responsible for maintaining wakefulness and alerting the cortex. When the RAS is inhibited fatigue is an outward manifestation, which could occur through lowered sensory input, decreased response to input (e.g., sensory deprivation, immobility, isolation) and reduced cortical activity through chronic stimulation such as would result from depression, anxiety, pain and narcotics. Astair (1987) links these mechanisms to a stress response, hence explaining how they contribute to fatigue in cancer patients. As well as physiological and situational factors, she postulates that psychological factors lead to chronic fatigue and labels anxiety, depression and crisis as energy-depleting states. The cognitive and affective elements within this theoretical model are so interwoven that they are difficult to separate. Psychological factors need separating out if the model is to be useful for treatment strategies.

Malaise: An Expression of Fatigue/Tiredness?

General malaise is said to indicate that an individual feels weak and tired and is unable to accomplish much. Kobashi et al. (1985), in a study of cancer patients treated with radiotherapy, found that malaise was highly correlated with "feeling ill, tired, not well and being inactive". Malaise is also used as a quality of life indicator in the fatigue literature (Hürny and Bernhard 1993). In our study, the German word "*Unwohlsein*" was used; Swiss people from the German-speaking part of Switzerland do not use the word malaise, as it is rooted in the French language. Respondents in this study perceived malaise in various ways. Some spoke of it in terms of "feeling nauseated," while others referred to it as a general feeling of "ill-being." They did not mention any feeling of tiredness in association with it. Only two of the 20 cancer patients felt that they experienced malaise. The same use of the concept malaise was apparent in the responses from the healthy individuals. Only two individuals mentioned malaise (*Unwohlsein*); the others denied it or gave unclear responses. This suggests that malaise in the German language and culture is better used as a measure of a wellness–illness dimension, rather than as a measure of tiredness.

Weakness: The Same as Tiredness?

Current research in fatigue recognizes the need to define the concept of weakness (Winningham et al. 1994; Piper and Lindsey 1989), and in particular to establish whether there is a difference between weakness and tiredness. In our study, general weakness was defined as an anticipatory, subjective sensation of difficulty in initiating a certain activity. It represents the definition used in the syndrome of asthenia, which does not include any localized or regional weakness resulting from neurological or muscle disorders (Bruera 1988). This implies that there is a voluntary component to fatigue, since an individual can still push him- or herself to perform certain tasks. When the word weakness is used to describe a symptom of neurological syndromes, on the other hand, there is no voluntary component in the performance of activities (Gordon 1986). In this study it was on these grounds that weakness resulting from neurological damage was differentiated from weakness associated with normal neurological function.

In this study cancer patients reported weakness spontaneously in the context of tiredness; it was in fact one of the three most frequently mentioned expressions of tiredness, together with feeling unusually tired and decreased physical performance. Whereas decreased physical performance could be a consequence of tiredness, however, it is more difficult to disentangle the concept of weakness from feelings of unusual tiredness. A possible solution is to use the notion of a voluntary component to distinguish the meaning of the two concepts, even though it leaves a problem unsolved: decreased physical performance might limit the capacity to overcome tiredness. For, if one argues that tiredness is a consequence of decreased physical performance it leads to a vicious circle within all of the four most frequently mentioned expressions of physical fatigue/tiredness: unusual tiredness leads to decreased physical performance (or vice versa), decreased physical performance leads to weakness (or vice versa), weakness leads to an unusual need for rest (or vice versa). What then needs to be explained, for treatment purposes, is how this vicious circle could be broken, or at least slowed down, by either physical or emotional interventions. In an exploratory study, breast cancer patients receiving chemotherapy who participated in a supervised aerobic interval training exercise program showed an improvement in mood that included corresponding changes in the perception of fatigue (MacVicar and Winningham 1986). But the type of fatigue in the breast cancer patients might have been different from the fatigue felt by patients with advanced small cell lung cancer who are not receiving antineoplastic treatment. This hypothesis is supported by a report from St. Pierre and Kasper (1992), who suggests that exercise could increase feelings of fatigue through the effects of tumor necrosis factor on skeletal muscle in patients with certain types of advanced cancer. This emphasizes the need to separate the voluntary components of fatigue from the physical components.

Data from this interview study suggest that weakness (differentiated from weakness caused from neurological damage) is inherent in the tiredness/fatigue felt by cancer patients. This notion is supported by the different forms taken by weakness in healthy individuals, since their tiredness was not associated with weakness: 12 of the 20 healthy individuals specifically said that their tiredness was not weakness, and for the other eight individuals it was unclear.

Difference in Perception of Fatigue/Tiredness Between Healthy Individuals and Cancer Patients

The healthy individuals in this study also reported physical, affective and cognitive expressions of tiredness, but perceived them on different grounds. Cancer patients spoke about a chronic, unpleasant, distressing, life- and activity-limiting tiredness throughout the day, whereas the healthy individuals, in general, reported tiredness as a pleasant, acute, normal, regulating phenomenon, which helped them to schedule their daily rhythm and which disappeared after a good night's sleep. This relationship of tiredness to circadian rhythm was described in a study comparing fatigue profiles of healthy individuals with those who had either cancer or inflammatory bowel disease (Glaus 1993). Many of the healthy individuals perceived it as pleasant sign, indicating that it was time to relax, most of them relating it to the effects of work or to extra physical exercise. Whereas in cancer patients tiredness was more a "whole-body" feeling, in healthy individuals tiredness was experienced locally in those parts of the body that were involved in work. Sleepiness in the healthy persons was experienced as a period of relaxation after work or during a break, whereas in cancer patients sleepiness was more a general, increased need for sleep or a feeling of "tiredness in the head" (mentally tired). Healthy persons did report depressive feelings, loss of energy or decreased activity as well as cognitive deficiencies, but these usually disappeared after rest. This recovery after rest was not necessarily experienced by the cancer patients. As described above, malaise was not understood as tiredness in either of the groups, while weakness was only experienced by cancer patients. The results therefore suggest that tiredness in our sample of cancer patients represents an unusual tiredness with distressing correlates, while tiredness in healthy people is perceived as a normal regulating phenomenon. Therefore, while for both groups the expression of tiredness occurs on physical, affective and cognitive levels, the origins of its cause led to very different meanings, experiences and impact for each group.

Different Types of Fatigue/Tiredness

Building a Framework of Physical, Affective and Cognitive Categories

The research question "what is it, what does it feel like," generated categories that represent fatigue/tiredness as an experience of the whole person; it includes both body and mind. The analysis illustrates expressions of tiredness, addressing the experience as lived but not the consequences of tiredness or the causes. It produced three categories of physical, affective, and cognitive fatigue/tiredness. A similar classification system was constructed by Kobashi et al. (1985) in his design of an instrument to measure feelings of malaise in patients with radiotherapy. It had four scales: a physical fatigue scale, a men-

Table 7. Steps in the production of fatigue/tiredness in cancer patients

Step	Conditioning factors
1. Nociception	Specificity: physical type, stage of cancer, cytokines, biochemical factors, metabolic disorders, treatment, energy transformation patterns, symptoms. Psychological, social: reactions, coping (anxiety, depression, fear, isolation)
2. Perception	Decreasing inhibitory pathways, threshold (affective state, coping mechanisms social support network, beliefs, personality, general well-being)
3. Expression	At physical, affective and cognitive level

tal fatigue scale, a malaise scale and a psychological complaint scale. Yoshitake (1971) validated a 30-item fatigue-symptom checklist in a healthy working population in Japan and divided it into three similar categories of "dull sleepy factors," "decline of working motivation" and "projection of fatigue in some part of the body," which partially fits in with the categorization of fatigue into physical, affective, and cognitive expressions.

A way of underpinning a model of physical, affective and cognitive fatigue/tiredness as an expression is to use the way Bruera (1994) explains pain, which could explain the production of fatigue/tiredness in the form of steps (Table 7). The production of pain is described in three steps: nociception, perception, and expression. The same steps could be used to explain the production of tiredness. Nociception might be specifically cancer related in origin and represent the biochemical, pathophysiological causes of tiredness. The nociceptors could be explained as cytokines, regulated by the type and stage of disease, or as metabolic disorders accompanying cancer disease, as treatment-related causes, as nutritional deficits arising from a disrupted energy transformation process and further causes. Nociceptors could also be explained as psychological causes such as depression, fear and anxiety. These nociceptors might correspond primarily with physical and cognitive expressions of tiredness. Perception of fatigue may vary according to individual personality, a person's feeling of vulnerability, ways of coping with threat, level of general well-being and the person's social support network, which might then influence (decrease or increase) inhibitory pathways or modulate threshold. Perception might primarily correspond with the affective expression of tiredness. Expression may vary according to the personality and hence determine physical, affective or cognitive level. Since it is not yet possible to measure fatigue/tiredness at a cortical level, any assessment has to be based on the patient's expression of fatigue/tiredness. As this is influenced by factors that modulate the levels of nociception, perception and expression, research needs to focus on measurement and interventions that work at these different levels.

Linguistic Digression on Names for Fatigue/Tiredness in the Two Study Samples

An analysis was undertaken to evaluate the subjects' wording when they reported the phenomenon. It can, however, be recognized that healthy people associate tiredness more with humorous expressions (e.g., "it's time to hit the sack"). These words give the idea that tiredness is a normal phenomenon in life, which indicates feeling "finished, at zero, flat, time to go to bed" (Table 5). Cancer patients used no humorous expressions; rather, they included loss of strength, uncertainty, unwellness, and changes in mood, and they had more difficulty finding any words other than "simply tired" (Table 3). It is possible that the words used by the cancer patients are a mixture of physical and affective expressions of fatigue/tiredness, whereas in healthy people they may only represent physical expressions.

Reliability and Validity

In this study the use of unstructured interviews, with tape recording and transcription of each, allowed collection of "the native's view" without major distortion of data, which in itself contributes to validity as it demonstrates credibility. Content analysis, the picking out of themes and grouping them into categories, on the other hand, is subject to interpretation. To reduce possible bias, constant comparison was used to improve validity. Strict application of constant comparison was difficult, however, because there was a large data set, making it difficult to cope with the analysis.

As data triangulation improves credibility, three approaches were used. Multiple key informants were interviewed on the same topic, a second investigator judged the assignment of themes/categories to the significant passages in the interviews (interrater reliability) and multiple theoretical perspectives were used to interpret the data.

Transferability, which equates with generalizability of the quantitative approach (Polit and Hungler 1993), was achieved through the collection of life experiences from a sample of subjects who represent the population in question. Cancer patients were all experts on the phenomenon under investigation. However, a group of patients with different types and stages of cancer or who were all undergoing the same treatment might have yielded different results. The only variables used to select the sample (cancer patients and healthy individuals) were age and gender. Mean age turned out to be lower in the healthy population (Table 1) and could account for some of the difference between the ill and the healthy. Data saturation in both groups suggested that the data could be generalized to both groups under investigation.

Dependability, which is reflected in the stability of data over time and conditions, was not addressed in this study, as interviews were conducted on only one occasion for each subject. Confirmability, objectivity or neutrality of the data was supported through the agreement with the coding frame by a second researcher. The high percentage of agreement between the two researchers assures reliability of the identification of the themes but does not guarantee content validity, since the second researcher was acquainted with the coding frame.

Frequencies cannot be interpreted in the same way as they are in quantitative studies because of imprecise sampling (Polit and Hungler 1993). Quasi-statistics may allow conclusions if a phenomenon either never or always occurs, such as weakness and malaise in this study. Frequencies did show dominance in certain themes, which is interesting for theory development; however the occurrence of other, less frequent codes cannot be neglected, as the frequency and depth of data are both important.

Conclusions and Future Research Directions

The results of this study show differences between cancer patients and healthy individuals in the characteristics of their experience of fatigue/tiredness as lived. This finding is important for future research in cancer-related assessment of this distressing symptom, since it suggests the need to distinguish between fatigue/tiredness as distress and fatigue/tiredness as a normal life experience. The emerging concepts fit a theoretical framework according to which fatigue/tiredness is broken down into expressions of physical, affective and cognitive fatigue/tiredness. It has been argued that nociception, perception and expression could be considered as steps in the development of fatigue/tiredness. A theoretical framework that is able to represent the different forms in which fatigue in cancer patients is expressed would generate new research strategies, leading to new methods of assessment and treatment.

Further research is now needed to confirm the emergent hypothesis. Given that the concept remains robust, available measurement instruments must be studied to compare their content with the findings of this study. If the present instruments are not adequate to them, further instruments could then be developed to assess the physical, affective and cognitive components of fatigue. Because of its naturalistic nature, the results of our study cannot be generalized to a specific cancer population. It will be necessary to extend validation to include a large cancer patient sample. The controlling variables that need to be considered in any further research include nociceptor-related factors, such as type and stage of the disease, treatment patterns, symptoms and psychological aspects, such as anxiety and depression.

To develop nursing strategies that target fatigue/tiredness, it is particularly important that the three types of fatigue/tiredness identified be differentiated. It has also been argued that decreased physical performance, weakness, extreme tiredness, increased need for rest, inactivity, increased need for sleep, sadness or cognitive problems can fuse into a vicious circle. Further research is thus also needed to detect measures that could cause a break in this cycle. As nurses cope with deficits related to daily activities and with impaired quality of life, fatigue/tiredness research represents a real challenge for nursing.

References

Astair J (1987) Fatigue in the cancer patients: a conceptual approach to a clinical problem. Oncol Nurs Forum 14 (6):25–30

Baker C, Wuest J, Stern P (1992) Method slurring: the grounded theory/phenomenology example. J Adv Nurs 17:1355–1360

Bruera E (1988) Asthenia in patients with advanced cancer. J Pain Symptom Manage 18 (1):81–87

Bruera E (1994) New developments in the assessment of pain in cancer patients. Support Care Cancer 2:312–318

Chalmers AF (1982) What is this thing called science? Open University Press, Buckingham

Chenitz WC (1994) Surfacing nursing process: a method for generating nursing theory from practice. J Adv Nurs 9:205–215

Cimprich B (1992) A theoretical perspective on attention and patient education. Adv Nurs Sci 14 (3):39–51

Clarke L (1995) Nursing research: science, visions and telling stories. J Adv Nurs 21:584–593

Field P, Morse J (1994) Nursing research: the application of qualitative approaches. Chapmann and Hall, Norwich

Gibson H, Edwards R (1985) Muscular exercise and fatigue. Sports Med 2:121

Glaser B (1978) Theoretical sensitivity. Sociological Press, Mill Valley

Glaser B, Strauss A (1967) The discovery of grounded theory: strategies for qualitative research. Aldine, New York

Glaus A (1993) Assessment of fatigue in cancer and non-cancer patients and in healthy individuals. Support Care Cancer 1:305–315

Gordon M (1986) Differential diagnosis of weakness: a common geriatric symptom. Geriatrics 41:75–79

Grandjean E (1970) Fatigue. Am Ind Hyg Assoc J 31:401–411

Harris M (1968) The rise of anthropological theory. Crowell, New York

Hürny C, Bernhard J (1993) "Fatigue and malaise" as a quality of life indicator in small-cell lung cancer patients. Support Care Cancer 1:316–320

Irvine D, Vincent L, Graydon J (1994) The prevalence and correlates of fatigue in patients receiving treatment with chemotherapy and radiotherapy. Cancer Nurs 17 (5):367–378

Kobashi J, Hanewald G, Van Dam F (1985) Assessment of malaise in cancer patients treated with radiotherapy. Cancer Nursing 8 (6):306–313

Lincoln YS, Guba EG (1985), Naturalistic inquiry. Sage, Newbury Park

MacVicar MG, Winningham ML (1986) Promoting the functional capacity of cancer patients. Cancer Bull 38:235–239

Melia KM (1992) Tell it as it is – qualitative methodology and nursing research: understanding the student nurses' world. J Adv Nurs 12:331–337

Miles M, Huberman A (1984) Qualitative data analysis: a source book of new methods. Sage, Beverly Hills

Morant R (1991) Asthenia in cancer patients – a double edged inflammatory response against the tumour? J Palliat Care 7:22–24

Morse J (1991) Qualitative nursing research: a free-for-all? In: Morse J (ed) Qualitative nursing research: a contemporary dialogue. Sage, Newbury

Omery A (1983) Phenomenology. a method for nursing research. Adv Nurs Sci 5 (2):49–63)

Oppenheim AN (1992) Questionnaire, design, interviewing and attitude measurement. Pinter, London

Piper B (1993) Fatigue. In: Carrieri V, Lindsey A, West C (eds) Pathophysiological phenomena in nursing, human response to illness. Saunders, Philadelphia, pp 279–302

Piper B, Lindsey A (1989) Development of an instrument to measure the subjective dimension of fatigue. In: Funk S, Tornquist E (eds) Key aspects of comfort. Springer, Berlin Heidelberg New York, pp 199–208

Piper B, Rieger P (1989) Recent advances in the management of biotherapy-related side effects: fatigue. Oncol Nurs Forum [Suppl] 16 (6):27–34

Polit D, Hungler B (1993) Essentials of nursing research. Lippincott, Philadelphia
Schag C, Heinrich R, Ganz P (1984) Karnofsky performance status revisited: reliability, validity and guidelines. J Clin Oncol 2 (3):187–193
St Pierre B, Kasper CE (1992) Fatigue mechanisms in patients with cancer: effects of tumor necrosis factor and exercise on skeletal muscle. Oncol Nurs Forum 19:419–425
Weis E (1990) PONS Kompaktwörterbuch. Klett, Stuttgart
Winningham M, Nail L, Barton Burke M, et al (1994) Fatigue and the cancer experience: the state of the knowledge. Oncol Nurs Forum 21 (1):23–36
World Health Organisation (1990) Cancer pain relief and palliative care. WHO, Geneva (Technical report series 804)
Yoshitake H (1971) Relations between the symptoms and feelings of fatigue. Ergonomics 14 (1):175–186

Construction of a New Fatigue Assessment Questionnaire

Introduction

Current literature shows that there is a gap in our knowledge about how tiredness/fatigue in cancer patients should be defined and measured. Existing fatigue-related research in cancer patients shows conceptual and measurement differences (Piper 1993). There is no continuum of tiredness/fatigue in universal use. What do patients mean if they fill in a visual analogue scale indicating that they feel "very tired"? Is it an indicator of general well-being, and thus an estimate of general quality of life (Hürny and Bernhard 1993)? Most articles written by English authors use the word fatigue to identify extreme tiredness. It could be said that in the English language, tiredness that is perceived as unusual, continuing distress is fatigue rather than tiredness. In the German language, tiredness (*Müdigkeit*) is not primarily a term for distress attributed to disease or unusual effort. But tiredness becomes a distressing phenomenon when it no longer regulates a healthy balance between rest and activity but represents unusual, abnormal or excessive whole-body tiredness that is disproportionate to or unrelated to activity or excessive exertion (Piper 1993). As there is no word for fatigue in the German language, the definition "extreme, unusual tiredness" (in German: *extreme, unübliche Müdigkeit*), is used to explain the term "fatigue." This clarification is needed to ensure that future fatigue research conducted in German-speaking countries can be compared with such research carried out elsewhere.

The qualitative exploration of the experience of the concept fatigue in cancer patients and healthy individuals in the previous chapter has given us an insight into the multidimensionality of this phenomenon. It was concluded that it was expressed at physical, affective and cognitive levels and that there was a distinct difference between fatigue in cancer patients and fatigue in healthy individuals. The interviews yielded specific descriptors with which cancer patients name their fatigue. It is the aim of this chapter to compare these identified descriptors from the last chapter with those used in currently available measurement instruments. The applicability of the available instruments for further epidemiological fatigue research in cancer patients will be discussed. The development of the new Fatigue Assessment Questionnaire (FAQ) will be justified, and the process of questionnaire development will be described.

Review of Different Types of Quality of Life Measurement Instruments Incorporating Assessment of Fatigue or Tiredness

References cited in the review are based on Medline literature searches with CD ROM over the period of 1988–1995. Further literature was detected by searching for studies in which fatigue was assessed as part of quality of life research.

Fatigue/tiredness is a complex phenomenon, which is often incorporated into tools that measure a broader set of concepts. Few tools are constructed to measure fatigue per se. According to their aim and application, they address different underlying concepts and aspects of fatigue (McNair and Lorr 1971; Piper and Lindsey 1989; Kobashi and Hanewald 1985; Hürny and Bernhard 1993). Items in existing tools seem mainly to be derived from clinical experience and the existing literature.

The Vigor/Fatigue Subscale of the Profile of Mood States

The original purpose of the Profile of Mood States (POMS; McNair and Lorr 1971) is the assessment of mood states in different populations. A subscale of this validated and reliability-tested instrument includes fatigue, with the items worn out, listless, fatigued, exhausted, sluggish, weary and bushed, in order to assess a mood of weariness, inertia and low energy level. The adjectives are rated by the respondents on a five-point scale (0–4) from not at all, through a little, moderately, and quite a bit, to extremely (McNair and Lorr 1971). Several time sets have been tested. However, most of the data reported are based on a one-week period (McNair and Lorr 1971). Interestingly, the item tired was dropped during the instrument development phase, as tired and fatigued seemed to be a doublet in earlier tests. As this instrument is primarily used to assess mood disturbances, it might not represent symptoms of fatigue caused mainly by physical disease, such as cancer. Weakness and malaise, which are probably more somatic expressions of fatigue, are also not addressed. However, self-rated fatigue intensity has been shown to correlate significantly with the scores on the POMS subscale for fatigue–inertia assessment (Blesch and Paice 1991). The same was true for the other subscale, concerning tension–anxiety, depression–dejection, anger–hostility and confusion–bewilderment (Blesch and Paice 1991). These findings support the idea that physical and psychological expressions of the cancer experience may be difficult to disentangle. Furthermore, it is unclear whether psychological distress is a consequence of tiredness or whether tiredness is an expression of emotional distress.

The question remains as to whether there is an emotional component of fatigue that differs from the physical sensation component. Cella and Orofiamma (1987) used the POMS instrument to explore the relationship between psychological distress, extent of disease, and performance status in 304 cancer patients. Regression analysis indicated that fatigue and vigor were most highly related to the covariates in the model, with total mood disturbance and confusion close behind. The question of whether fatigue and vigor were the most "physical" symptoms (physical fatigue components) was raised, and also whether they accounted for the association of performance status with the extent of disease. Total mood disturbance scores rose in a linear fashion, with greater impairment in performance status and with tension, vigor and fatigue subtests explaining most of this effect. Concerning tension, it could be seen as a response to stress, which leads to tiredness and so contributes to loss of vigor and is hence expressed as fatigue.

The primary purpose of the POMS instrument appears to be the assessment of mood states in different populations, with a main focus on fatigue originating in mood disturbances. The validity and reliability of this subscale, taken out of the context of the whole POMS instrument, would need further reliability testing when used in a physically ill population. The whole instrument, with 65 items, might be too long and unspecific to be used as a viable tool in a cancer patient population with restricted energy. However, the tension–anxiety and the vigor–fatigue subscales address fatigue from the perspective of mood, which is of high interest if fatigue in cancer patients is being hypothesized as both an emotional and a physical experience.

The C30 Quality of Life Questionnaire (EORTC)

The European Organization for Research and Treatment of Cancer (EORTC) has developed a Core Quality of Life Questionnaire to assess quality of life in cancer patients (Aaronson and Ahmedzai 1993). One subscale of this questionnaire contains five questions concerning fatigue and malaise, in a Likert format, range 1–4. Patients answer the questions in relation to the past week. This reliability- and validity-tested instrument was used in a study which showed that fatigue and malaise were the most prominent symptoms for six months after diagnosis and during cytotoxic treatment of small cell lung cancer patients. The authors concluded that fatigue and malaise can be used as an indicator of quality of life in this patient population and that the positive correlations of fatigue with psychological distress, role functioning, restriction of social activity and impaired general well-being were more likely to be based on the consequences of fatigue and malaise (Hürny and Bernhard 1993).

The five items addressed in this questionnaire are: (1) have you felt weak? (2) physically well? (3) ill? (4) tired? and (5) did you need rest? (during the past week). These items appear to be addressing the state of general well-being (since the instrument is a quality of life questionnaire) and include the illness–wellness continuum, which could be interpreted as a measurement of malaise. Weakness and tiredness are also included, and there seems to be an emphasis on these through the assessment of the need for rest. These items are based on the theory that fatigue and malaise are caused by the disease process, its treatment, and psychological distress, thus representing a multidimensional concept (Hürny and Bernhard 1993). However, it seems that the components being measured refer more to physical tiredness than to fatigue as a mood state. The subscale of this tool is likely to measure fatigue from a physical perspective. Items related to mood are integrated into other parts of the questionnaire. The use of this subscale, if taken out of the context of the entire EORTC Quality of Life Questionnaire, would need further validity and reliability testing. The application of the entire, multidimensional quality of life questionnaire with its 42 items would be too broad and extensive for the purpose of exploring fatigue specifically in cancer patients.

Fatigue/Tiredness in a Selection of Quality of Life Questionnaires and Indexes of Abilities, Functional Living, Performance, and Activity

A very wide variety of indexes are being used today to assess quality of life or influencing factors for different purposes. An ability index can be helpful in the assessment of impairment of daily living. As an example, the ability index of Izak and Medalie reflects subjective reactions, working abilities and social adjustment (Izak and Medalie 1971). Fatigue is not mentioned in this index, even though many of the items could be used as indicators of fatigue or the consequences of fatigue. To know more about the impact of fatigue, questions would need to include such phrases as "How much has fatigue impaired your ability to work?" The question remains whether impairment of abilities can be strictly related to fatigue and whether the causes of such impairment can be discriminated from fatigue.

A functional living index measures factors contributing to overall functional living. Examples of two such indexes are the Functional Living Index and the Functional Assessment of Cancer Therapy tool. The Functional Living Index–Cancer, or FLIC (Schipper and Clinch 1984), measures distinct physical, emotional, and social factors. This instrument does not mention tiredness or fatigue, but many of the items, again, could be seen as consequences of fatigue. The Functional Assessment of Cancer Therapy Tool (FACT; Cella 1990) seems to include fatigue with the item "lack of energy." The item "forced to spend time in bed" could also be interpreted as an indicator of fatigue. While a functional or ability index is likely to be influenced by fatigue, it does necessarily account for the possible consequences of fatigue. The question that emerges is, "What kind of fatigue reduces abilities and functionality?" Is it physical tiredness, weakness, or tiredness as a mood state?

The Breast Cancer Chemotherapy Questionnaire (Levin and Guyatt 1988) includes fatigue with the items "felt low in energy" and "felt tired or fatigued while hurrying" (during the last 2 weeks). A further item looks at "problems with fatigue or tiredness which limited usual social activities." This item pays regard to the impact or consequences of fatigue. However, the impact might be multicausal. The tool is especially constructed for breast cancer patients under chemotherapy and not for a general cancer population.

The Cancer Rehabilitation Evaluation System (CARES; CARES Consultants 1988) includes fatigue, with the items "I do not have the energy I used to," "feel tired after chemotherapy," "feel tired after radiotherapy" (past month, including today). This system compares actual fatigue perception in comparison with the patient's earlier state and involves differentiation of therapy-induced fatigue.

The Quality of Life Index devised by Padilla asks about items related to general physical conditions, important human activities and general quality of life aspects (Padilla and Presant 1983). Under physical condition it asks, "How much strength do you feel" (LASA, from none to normal). Impaired strength could be interpreted as fatigue or weakness.

The Karnofsky Performance Index (KPI) and the World Health Organisation (Zubrod) scales are commonly used as proxy measures of performance and quality of life. Their historical relevance and current high frequency of usage, despite their unidimensionality, are remarkable. They represent an index of activity from normal to dead (Karnofsky and Abelmann 1948) and from normal to unable to get out of bed (Zubrod and Schneidermann 1960). Performance could be significantly correlated with fatigue but might still arise from different sources. The KPI has been tested against the Cancer Inventory of Problem Situations (CIPS) concerning the components "self-care," "daily activity," "work" and "evidence of disease." The CIPS is a self-administered instrument that assesses the type and severity of problems confronted by cancer patients (Heinrich and Schag 1983). One item of the "evidence of disease-component" was described as "I do not have the energy I used to." In this study, patients who obtained the highest Karnofsky Performance Scores when rated by health care professionals rated themselves as having some impairment, and 74% had reduced energy (Schag and Heinrich 1984). While statistically the KPI is a reliable instrument, it appears that the absence of guidelines for its use has created a certain degree of unreliability. In the last study mentioned, the KPI was shown to have very good interrater reliability (Schag and Heinrich 1984). However, as fatigue is not necessarily a visible expression, specific assessment by the patients themselves seems needed. Again questions emerge: Why is performance impaired? Why does fatigue as a performance-impairing factor appear? And is it a physical cause or a mood state, or both?

Review of Symptom Distress Scales

Symptoms can be caused by the disease itself or by its treatment. Scales have been widely used in the assessment of symptom distress. Fatigue as a form of distress is incorporated in few of them. The symptom distress scale developed by McCorkle and Young (1978) includes ten symptoms, one of which is fatigue. Patients are asked to put a circle around the number (ranging from 1 to 5, indicating "could not feel more tired" to "I am not tired at all") that most closely represents how they perceive their distress at a specific moment of the day.

Tiredness is defined as an unspecific state, which could be part of normal life. Holmes developed and validated a measurement instrument to assess symptom distress in cancer patients; this had 11 items and used a linear analogue scale. Scores for each symptom were obtained by simple measurement (in millimeters), with a value of 100 assigned to the end of the scale, indicating "normality" or the absence of distress; while zero represented extreme distress and higher scores indicated less distress from individual items (Holmes 1991). The item "fatigue" was described as "could not feel more tired" at one end and as "I do not feel tired at all" at the other end. In a study using this instrument in 51 chemotherapy and radiotherapy patients, the symptom "tiredness" was recognized as the cause of the highest distress (significant distress defined as arbitrary cut-off point of 50 mm), followed by "appearance," "mood," and "concentration" (Holmes 1991). Tiredness, again, was not further defined.

Another example of a symptom assessment scale is the Edmonton Symptom Assessment Scale, which was developed for daily use in a palliative care population. It consists of nine visual analogue scales for nine different symptoms (Bruera 1991). Interestingly, fatigue is not included as a symptom, even though its prevalence is thought to be high in patients with advanced neoplastic disease. The dimensions of well-being, drowsiness, depression, and activity are included and could be seen as indicators or consequences of fatigue. It seems that fatigue is only slowly being recognized and acknowledged as a symptom in its own right. Another explanation would be that it has been difficult to influence this kind of distress and therefore a nihilistic attitude prevails.

Symptom distress scales measure tiredness unidimensionally and give information about the intensity and impact of tiredness. However, the use of such a scale does not in itself explain what the symptom represents. Is it a symptom that expresses physical distress or a mood state, or both? Furthermore, we need a separate definition of tiredness meaning cancer-specific tiredness, as this might not be comparable to the tiredness experienced by healthy individuals.

Review of Fatigue-Specific Measurement Instruments

The Rhoten Fatigue Scale

Specific scales to measure fatigue specifically have also been developed. The Rhoten Fatigue Scale is a 10-point subjective rating of fatigue severity, ranging from "not tired, full of energy, peppy" (0), to total "exhaustion" (10). This self-assessment scale was used to quantify fatigue in postsurgical patients, and the results were compared with those obtained with an observation checklist used concurrently by the caregivers to document visible signs of fatigue (Rhoten 1982). It is doubtful whether subjective, self-reported fatigue can be compared with observations from caregivers, as the latter might impose their own judgement and visible signs might reflect responses to other distress. As subjectivity of fatigue requires self-assessment, measurement by caregivers does not appear to have adequate validity. Furthermore, the continuum of tiredness in postsurgical patients is likely to be different from that in a general cancer population.

The Piper Fatigue Scale

The Piper Fatigue Scale measures four dimensions of subjective fatigue, temporal, affective, sensory and severity (among these areas are 41 visual analogue scale items that yield a total fatigue score) plus three open-ended items, addressing perceived cause, relief measures and associated symptoms (Piper 1992). Fatigue is not further defined as a symptom, but its impact on daily living and possible indicators are assessed. Physical functioning and emotional feelings, possible indicators of fatigue, are addressed. This tool aims at measuring fatigue as a physical state and as mood state at the time of measurement. It is developed from an underlying framework of fatigue, which is multidimensional (Piper and Lindsey 1989). This tool measures intensity, temporal properties and distress; however, a cancer-specific fatigue continuum is not defined. It can offer the possibility of recognizing indicators and consequences of fatigue and allows calculation of total fatigue scores. It seems to be the most comprehensive fatigue measurement tool presently available. The design and selection of the items of the tool were guided by clinical experience and by the literature on symptom measurement, and on measurement of fatigue and pain in particular (Piper and Lindsey 1989). It has been successfully tested for validity and reliability (Piper 1992). What patients mean if they rate feelings of fatigue on the visual analogue scale, however, remains unclear. As the instrument is extensive, its use could be helpful in individual assessment and care planning, rather than in large epidemiological studies. A shortened version (20 items) of this scale is currently being tested.

Linear Fatigue Assessment Scales

A multiple Linear Analogue Fatigue Scale (LAFS) has been constructed to assess fatigue in cancer patients and in healthy individuals over a daily period. The scales range from "I do not feel tired at all" to "I feel totally exhausted." Measurements were performed four times on each test day, at 0700, 1200, 1700 and 2100 hours. The scale was able to detect specific fatigue profiles over a daily period in healthy persons and in cancer patients (Glaus 1993). This scale primarily quantifies fatigue but, through its repeated use over daily periods, also assesses the characteristic impact of fatigue in a diurnal rhythm. While healthy persons started their day with a minimum of fatigue and showed high fatigue levels after work in the evening, cancer patients were significantly more tired in the morning and stayed tired during the day, but were somewhat less tired in the evening. These profiles can give an impression of whether fatigue is a healthy, regulatory response or whether it is a distressing, permanent symptom. Like other instruments (McCorkle and Young 1978; Holmes 1991), it does not assess the severity, nature or perception of fatigue. The author got the impression that exhaustion was not the opposite of cancer-specific tiredness, but rather the opposite of "no tiredness in healthy individuals." This emphasizes that the "unusual tiredness" of cancer patients requires clarification of fatigue/tiredness as a concept.

Kobashi developed a tool with four visual analogue scales to investigate malaise in 95 cancer patients during radiotherapy treatment. The scales examined four components of fatigue. The first dealt with tiredness, with a scale anchored by "I did not feel tired yesterday" and "I felt very tired yesterday". The other scales' extremes were: "not active" and "very active"; "not ill" and "ill"; and "not well" and "well," always referring to the condition of the previous day. These four items were considered to indicate a general condition of loss of energy. The clinical observation that complaints expressing malaise of cancer patients may increase within a few weeks of radiotherapy was corroborated by a statistically significant increase in the scores on a scale containing these four simple items (Kobashi and Hanewald 1985). The scales address both the illness/wellness complex and the activity dimension, which are incorporated in some other tools but otherwise never measured as main components of fatigue. Only the subscale of the EORTC C30 Quality of Life Questionnaire, as described above, measures similar aspects, such as activity, illness/wellness, general well-being. It measures tiredness as a non-cancer-specific continuum and looks at related components, which could be expressions or indicators of fatigue.

Lastly, these two measurement tools show that a relationship could exist between fatigue, general well-being, activity, quality of life and disease, with its physical and behavioral consequences. However, the emotional dimension, such as the impact of sadness or anxiety on vigor and fatigue, is not addressed specifically. Neither the underlying sources or nature, nor the continuum of fatigue are defined in these instruments.

The Pearson-Byars Fatigue Feeling Checklist

The Pearson-Byars Fatigue Feeling Checklist was originally developed to measure tiredness in airmen (Pearson and Byars 1956). Individuals are asked to indicate their feelings six times a day. The items (phrases) range within a continuum from 1 (extremely peppy) to 10 (ready to drop). This instrument was created from a viewpoint of physiology, considering a healthy continuum extending from "feeling peppy and refreshed" to "feeling extremely tired" and "being ready to drop". The term "fatigue" is not used in this scale, which might represent the characteristic nature of tiredness in healthy military personnel. Tiredness, as assessed here, does not seem to be addressed as a mood state and is seen as something that can be resolved by rest, which (as clinically experienced) is not necessarily the case in cancer patients. The authors themselves question whether the checklist is unidimensional. It seems that it measures mainly the intensity of physical tiredness. Pathophysiological aspects of tiredness/fatigue are not the underlying hypothesis of this checklist. Weakness and malaise are not included. The application of the viewpoint of physiology in healthy individuals might not be appropriate to the investigation of fatigue in cancer patients. Nevertheless, the scale has been tested in several clinical studies, with comparable reliability and validity estimates (Freel and Hart 1977; Haylock and Hart 1979; Jamar 1989). The postwar phraseology from the 1950s has been described as possibly outdated and difficult for patients to understand today (Winningham and Nail 1994).

The Yoshitake Fatigue Symptom Checklist

Yoshitake developed a symptom checklist to analyze symptoms of fatigue. Thirty symptoms are divided into three categories: (A) "dull, sleepy factors," (B) "decline of working motivation," (C) "projection of fatigue in some part of the body." This subjective report by individuals was primarily constructed for industrial workers in Japan, which explains the choice of its items. It describes a variety of symptoms of fatigue and pays regard to both physical and psychological factors at work. It has been tested for validity and reliability (Yoshitake 1971). Some authors have used it with cancer patient populations (Haylock and Hart 1979; Piper and Lindsey 1989). This instrument has concurrently been tested in healthy individuals, cancer patients and noncancer patients (Glaus 1993). Category A symptoms (dull, sleepy factors) were the most frequent in all three subpopulations. A significant difference between the subpopulations was observed in category B (mental symptoms) and C (projections into the body). Selected symptoms with a significant difference between cancer patients and the other subjects were: having a husky voice, being unable to straighten up (posture), becoming weary while talking, feeling thirsty, being unsteady while talking, feeling constrained in breathing, being anxious about things, feeling ill. Fatigue was presented as "whole-body fatigue" in cancer patients, but as localized muscle fatigue in the healthy working population; this corresponded with an assessment of the spatial distribution of fatigue that was done concurrently in this study. Even though this instrument had to be translated from English (originally Japanese) into German and has a background of physiology (fatiguability in industrial workers), it still revealed some fatigue problems specific to cancer patients and distinguished between fatigue of healthy and diseased persons. This tool thus successfully distinguishes between physical, mental and psychological fatigue symptoms and their expression. However, it does not pay any regard to the intensity of fatigue, even though the frequency of symptoms of fatigue could be an expression of its severity. It is not cancer-specific and represents fatigue extensively from the viewpoint of physiology in a healthy working population, which might not allow for valid description of fatigue in cancer patients.

Justification for the Construction of a New Fatigue Assessment Questionnaire: Evaluating the Applicability of the Instruments Reviewed for Further Epidemiological Fatigue Research in Cancer Patients

Selection of a measurement instrument depends heavily on the purpose of measurement and on the population concerned. If fatigue/tiredness is assessed as one of several quality of life aspects or as one symptom among others, a quality of life questionnaire or symptom distress scale will be applicable. As our aim is to conduct further specific fatigue research, a quality of life questionnaire does not apply in this case. In the instruments reviewed above, tiredness/fatigue is addressed mainly as the expression of the consequences of fatigue (Izak and Medalie 1971; Padilla and Presant 1983; Schipper and Clinch 1984; Levin and Guyall 1988; CARES Consultants 1988; Cella 1990). These consequences could be attributed to causes other than tiredness. For the intended epidemiological fatigue research, the aim is to measure the actual experience of fatigue and not the consequences of fatigue.

The subscale on fatigue in the EORTC Q30 questionnaire includes four important, simple questions that address tiredness directly (Hürny and Bernhard 1993) and from a perspective of general well-being and quality of life. However, it does not address affective expressions of fatigue. The same attributes apply to the malaise measurement tool developed by Kobashi and Hanewald (1985). The content analysis of the study reported in the previous chapter revealed the need for multidimensional measurement on the physical as well as the affective and cognitive levels.

The POMS subscale on vigor/fatigue (McNair and Lorr 1971) has been used and proved to be useful in fatigue measurement in cancer patients. Items in this scale, however, are derived from sources other than cancer patients' experience. Its emphasis on mood reflects its primary purpose. Items concerning physical expression of tiredness are scarce, and therefore this subscale cannot be used for the measurement of multidimensional fatigue. Concerning validity and reliability, the entire instrument has been widely tested in populations other than cancer patients.

Many of the symptom distress scales include tiredness as a single-item question. This restricted approach measures one dimension of a type of symptom distress. The concept of unusual tiredness in cancer patients is not defined in this context. A defined visual analogue scale with a definition of a reliable, cancer-specific fatigue continuum is needed to quantify the construct and the distress it causes.

The performance indexes reviewed do not measure tiredness, but are rather indicators of general well-being and activity status. The Karnofsky Index, together with instructions for its use by caregivers, has been proven valid, indicating a correlation between tiredness and performance in cancer patients. It could be very useful in fatigue research as an external criterion variable. It could also help to distinguish between affective and physical expression of fatigue if the Karnofsky Index score (physical performance) were compared with levels of physical and affective fatigue.

The general fatigue measurement tools reviewed have been developed for specific purposes. Therefore, their underlying theoretical frameworks differ. Fatigue research in industrial workers is based on the concept of physiology and needs different wording to capture the impact of tiredness on productivity or effectiveness; the background of physiology represents a different concept from that used as a background to pathophysiology in disease. Fatigue in cancer has a different nature, source and impact: cancer patients might not feel "refreshed, peppy or full of energy" in the morning, in contrast to active airmen, who are supposed to feel like that after a period of rest (Pearson and Byars 1956). The question of whether fatigue is a sign of depression, as assessed with the POMS instrument (McNair and Lorr 1971), requires different parameters than if fatigue is considered to be a physical consequence of biochemical changes resulting from cancer disease. The content analysis of the previous study revealed at least partially different themes in cancer patients than are reflected in the items of these general fatigue measurement instruments designed for healthy populations.

The Piper Fatigue Scale, probably the most sophisticated modern fatigue measurement tool developed for cancer patients, which is grounded in a multidimensional framework, measures fatigue from different viewpoints, with an emphasis on consequences of fatigue. This instrument might be very helpful in assessing consequences of fatigue on activities of daily living in individuals affected and for individual care planning or development of coping strategies. It does not, however, include all the themes identified in the previous study. The scale on fatigue itself does not differentiate between normal and unusual tiredness. With its 42 items it would be an unnecessary burden on the patients, as the aim is epidemiological measurement of the fatigue experience only.

It can be concluded from the analysis that the underlying theory of the questionnaire, the population concerned, and the purpose of its use determine the selection of specific items or tools. None of these instruments fully corresponds to the descriptors identified in the previous study (see the chapter "A Qualitative Study to Explore the Concept of Fatigue/Tiredness in Cancer Patients and in Healthy Individuals"). In addition, they measure aspects that are outside the scope of the intended epidemiological research and represent an unnecessary burden on the patients, measure constructs other than the experience of fatigue, or lack a corresponding underlying multidimensional framework that would support content validity.

Validity and Reliability: Essentials of Fatigue Measurement

Most of the instruments reviewed have been validated and tested for reliability in some way. This does not necessarily mean that they would be valid and reliable if used in any further investigation with a different study population.

The use of one of these tools could involve the risk of excluding important questions because the theoretical framework of the new study poses different questions. It remains to be reflected whether the research question can be answered with the aid of such a tool, whether it is sensitive enough or whether important information about the population under investigation may remain undetected by an insensitive measure.

It could be tempting to select desired items or sets of items from previously validated tools, but this is not a valid practice (Cella 1990). Selected items could, nevertheless, be chosen and validated in new populations. Translation of international instruments into a different language would again require validity and reliability testing, to ensure adequate wording and due consideration for cultural differences. Reliability and validity of a measurement instrument must be established in order to ensure scientific research.

Reliability

A tool cannot be considered valid until it has demonstrated satisfactory reliability. Reliability has been defined as the degree of consistency with which the instrument measures the attribute (Polit and Hungler 1993). Scale reliability has also been described as the proportion of variance attributable to a true score of the latent variable (De Vellis 1991). The latent variable is the underlying phenomenon or construct that a scale is intended to reflect; that is to say it is the actual phenomenon of interest. Scale items are necessary because many constructs cannot be measured directly, being comparable indicators of the underlying construct. Scales are reliable to the extent that they are comprised of reliable items that share a common latent variable. A scale developed to measure a latent variable is intended to estimate its actual magnitude at the time of measurement for each person measured. This unobservable "actual magnitude" is the true score (De Vellis 1991).

Scale reliability is therefore the proportion of variance attributable to the true score of the latent variable. Variability in a set of items can either be due to actual variation across individuals in the construct that the scale is intended to measure (the true variation in the latent variability) or it can be due to error. Error may reflect any remaining or unshared variation in scale scores, for example, unclear wording or unintended double meaning.

Scale reliability is therefore reflected in internal consistency of the scale items. A scale is internally consistent to the extent that its items are highly intercorrelated, thus measuring the same thing, implying strong links between items and the latent variable (De Vellis 1991). Internal consistency reflects whether certain items within one test make a difference to the total of scores obtained.

One method of examining internal consistency is to calculate coefficient alpha, typically equated with Cronbach's coefficient alpha (Cronbach 1951), where all possible ways of dividing the measure into two halves are used. The total variation of item scores is divided into two components: the true scores (true difference in patients) and the score differences caused by everything but the true difference (error). Computing alpha partitions the total of variance among the set of items into true scores and error scores. The proportion of the true scores equals alpha, which equals 1 minus error variance. A value of 0.70 has been suggested by Nunnally (1978) as the lowest acceptable limit for alpha, while others have described values between 0.65 and 0.70 as acceptable minima, between 0.70 and 0.80 as respectable, and between 0.80 and 0.90 as very good. It has been cautioned that a long scale should be shortened if it yields values above 0.90, because the reliability of alpha increases with the number of items and longer scales have a narrower confidence interval than when alpha is computed for shorter scales (De Vellis 1991).

However, reliability cannot be assumed if Cronbach's alpha is high, as internal consistency alone cannot guarantee reliability. Replication of the relationship between items in a further test must be possible (Fox 1995). Apart from the number of items, sample size, the probability level set for detecting error, the difference that is considered significant, heterogeneity and other sources all have an influence. For the calculation of alpha for items with dichotomous answers, a special version of alpha, the Kuder-Richardson formula 20, has been suggested (Nunnally 1978).

Other types of reliability computation to examine internal consistency involve having the same people complete two separate versions of a scale or the same version on multiple occasions. If two parallel forms of a scale exist and all members of the study population complete both forms, correlation can be computed, reflecting the alternate forms' reliability. A reliability measure of this type is called split-half reliability and has the aim of eliminating bias from item order. Instruments may be split into "first half–last half" items or "odd–even" items, because several factors may influence the reliability of answers, such as fatigue towards the end of the instrument, better responses to the items as individuals go along (practice effect), failure to complete the entire set, or such things as changes in print quality of the questionnaire.

Stability of an instrument reflects how constant scores remain from one occasion to another. The assessment of stability through the procedure of test–retest, using the same instrument in two different occasions, can show reliability through computing of a reliability coefficient. This stability test seems appropriate for attributes with enduring characteristics. Its approach has disadvantages in fluctuating states. Fatigue is a fluctuating construct, and therefore stability of a fatigue measurement tool is difficult to assess by the test–retest method.

Interrater reliability, also called equivalence, refers to the association of two or more judges. This is an issue if observer-rated tests are used. In fatigue research this approach seems difficult, because the observation might capture responses to different things than the phenomenon of fatigue itself. The subjectivity of fatigue makes it difficult to assess by anyone other than the person under study.

Apart from internal consistency and stability, other factors might influence reliability. Clear definition of the role of the investigator and the responder during measurement and a standardized measurement procedure seem crucial.

Knowledge of reliability of the instrument is useful in the interpretation of research results. If data fail to support a research hypothesis, one explanation might be that the instrument used was not representative or was unreliable. Using an instrument without knowledge of its reliability is taking a huge gamble, as there is no way of telling how far the results can be trusted and there is a danger that the study results will have to be disregarded.

Validity

Even if an instrument has been shown to be reliable, this is no guarantee of its validity: high reliability of an instrument provides no evidence of its validity for an intended purpose. The measurement of an attribute of fatigue can be consistent, reliable and still not valid if the attribute does not really reflect fatigue, but something else. Validity refers to the degree to which an instrument measures what it is supposed to be measuring (Polit and Hungler 1993).

Validity for fatigue measurement is connected with the question of whether what we ask for and measure represents the phenomenon experienced by the patient. Content validity refers to the question as to whether the content area in a test is representative. This necessarily means that experts need to analyze and judge the item's adequacy. Concerning fatigue, indicators must first be defined to be used in a cancer patient population. The selection of items in existing fatigue measurement tools has mostly been guided by clinical experience, professional expertise, existing literature, and dictionaries (McNair and Lorr 1971; Piper 1992; Aaronson and Ahmedzai 1993). There seems to be a lack of grounded data on "what fatigue is" or "what it feels like" as described by cancer patients themselves. The qualitative research method used in the study reported above (previous chapter) appeared appropriate for this purpose, as the information presently available is based mainly on sources other than the actual patients. Such grounded data can either confirm items in specific tools or reveal that patients in "the real world" feel differently.

It might be assumed that the best experts to identify descriptors of fatigue in cancer patients would be cancer patients themselves. As content validity is more difficult to evaluate if the domain under investigation is poorly defined, it seems a high priority should be assigned to enlarging the body of knowledge by studying cancer patients' perception of fatigue with qualitative research methods. Comparison of the expression of fatigue between healthy persons and cancer patients could clarify differences between normal transitory tiredness and tiredness as continuing distress in cancer patients.

The establishment of available criteria with which the measures on the target instrument can be compared allows criterion-related validity assessment.

The relationship between the scores on the instrument and some external criterion can support validity. A validity coefficient is computed by using a mathematical formula that correlates the scores on the instrument with scores on the criterion variable (Polit and Hungler 1993). Another validated instrument could be used as an external criterion to examine the correlation between new tools and established instruments and show concurrent and convergent validity. Unfortunately, no fatigue measurement instrument is available in the German language to examine the correlation with a new instrument.

Construct validity refers to the degree to which an instrument measures the construct under investigation. In fatigue research, it seems difficult to establish construct validity of an instrument, because the concept of fatigue is poorly defined. An approach to support the degree of evidence of construct validity could be the "known groups technique" (De Vellis 1991), according to which different groups, such as healthy individuals and cancer patients, would be expected to differ on the critical attribute, and some group differences would be reflected in the scores. Construct validity can also be assessed by factor analysis. Factor analysis of a new instrument could be compared with factor analysis of established instruments: identification of different factors would provide evidence of discriminant validity or the opposite would provide evidence for convergent validity. Factor analysis can also provide validity information if a preconceived theoretical framework is consistent with the factor analytic solution.

Some further pragmatic aspects may determine the validity of an instrument. Completion of the investigation could be used as an eligibility criterion, and assessment at the end of the study, including drop-outs, is needed to evaluate feasibility. The method of data collection, for example, interview or self-report, might impose greater or less bias on sensitive items owing to aspects of confidentiality. Subject burden has to be considered, as fatigued cancer patients present a vulnerable population. Lengthy and time-consuming fatigue tools might lead to an increase in missing data, which has been described as a major problem with the analysis of quality of life data (Smith 1993). Determination of both the time span for which data are collected for a specific purpose and the time-point of measurement is crucial. Another analysis problem is that data from a fatigue measurement tool could be confounded by other factors. Their potential impact on the results must be delineated and the set of dependent variables, the criterion variables, must be clearly identified. Specification of details of procedures and classification of subjects into identifiable groups are critically important to the conclusions. Sample size requirements need to be considered if meaningful research data are to be generated.

An instrument is not validated per se, but rather the application of the instrument. If "truth" is to be established in science, it is imperative that the reliability and validity of any measurement instrument used are beyond all doubt.

Development of a Fatigue Assessment Questionnaire for Use in a General Cancer Patient Population: Methodology

The literature review showed that the available fatigue measurement instruments did not fit the intended research purpose of measuring the experience of fatigue epidemiologically in cancer patients. Some are developed for populations other than cancer patients, while others do not measure fatigue on its own or do not measure the experience, but rather the consequences, of fatigue. Valid information from cancer patients, which reflects the true experience of fatigue, is needed to develop a fatigue measurement tool for specific research purposes. The qualitative, grounded research approach of the study reported above (previous chapter) did reveal such information and generated knowledge concerning the experience of fatigue, and it now serves as a basis to substantiate or weaken items from existing tools and to direct the content of a new fatigue assessment questionnaire. The steps in its development are described in the last part of this chapter. They were carried out in accordance with the guidelines for scale development, as described by De Vellis (1991).

Step 1: Item Generation

A patient-as-expert approach was taken when 20 cancer patients with different types and stages of disease explained what they felt when they experienced tiredness/fatigue. The interviews were unstructured, with the aim of not imposing already existing descriptions. Only one leading question was asked, concerning occurrence of weakness and malaise, if this was not mentioned spontaneously in the interview. This was done because it remains unclear whether weakness and malaise are the same phenomena as tiredness. Data saturation was well achieved after 20 interviews. After transcription, the interviews were content analyzed (see previous chapter). Sixteen themes were recognized: decreased physical performance, weakness/no strength, unusual need for sleep, unusual tiredness, unusual need for rest, decreased motivation, need to force oneself to overcome inactivity, no energy, sadness, anxiety, no fighting spirit, lack of concentration, problems in thinking, mental tiredness ("tired in the head"), sleeping problems at night, malaise. Malaise was recognized by only two of 20 patients, while weakness was mentioned spontaneously by most of them (by 17 out of 20). These 16 themes were expert statements from the persons concerned and thus valid descriptions of tiredness in this general cancer population.

In the next step, it was necessary to determine whether these experiences were really different from the experiences of a healthy population. Twenty healthy individuals described their experience of tiredness with the same methods of data collection and analysis. Again, only one leading question was asked, concerning the occurrence of weakness and malaise, and only if these were not mentioned spontaneously in the interview. Data saturation was well achieved after 20 interviews (as described earlier). Sixteen partially different themes were recognized: tiredness after a day's work (diurnal, as rhythmic normality), tiredness as a pleasant phenomenon (after exercise), wishing to go to bed (or to lie down, to rest, be silent), becoming slower, having heavy limbs, feeling exhausted (or worn-out, unable do any more), loss of energy, feeling depressive, wanting to withdraw, feeling impatient, loss of concentration (or forgetting easily, loss of attentiveness), difficulty in speaking, sleepiness, thoughts going around in the head, wishing to switch off, malaise. Malaise was experienced by only two of the 20 healthy individuals, and weakness was experienced by none of them.

Step 2: Reduction of Redundant Items

The items should capture the essence of the construct fatigue/tiredness and reflect overt manifestations of this latent variable. The scale's purpose was to measure these manifestations. It proved possible to reduce the total of 31 items from the two study subpopulations to a total of 22 items. This was due to overlapping items in the two groups (sadness, loss of interest, need for rest, malaise). Problems with thinking, speaking, and feeling "tired in the head" (mentally tired) were summarized under difficulties in concentrating. Loss of fighting spirit and decreased motivation were summarized under the item loss of interest (the word motivation was considered difficult to understand by the population under study). Tiredness after a working day and pleasant tiredness after physical exercise were pooled owing to their common nature.

Reduction of redundancy here meant the exclusion of items that were similar, unclear or seemingly irrelevant. The extraction of the items from interviews with the patients concerned supported validity in most of them. The length of the questionnaire had to be considered. The shorter a scale, the less burden it puts on respondents. Nevertheless, brevity tends to reduce reliability, and the optimal trade-off between brevity and reliability had to be considered (De Vellis 1991).

Step 3: Building Categories of Themes/Items

During content analysis of the interviews and identification of expressions and descriptions of tiredness, the emerging themes increasingly seemed to fit into three categories of physical, affective and cognitive expression of fatigue (see previous chapter). The current literature seems to use items derived from physical, or affective or cognitive origin, but only the measurement tool developed by Yoshitake (1971) has made a distinction between "dull sleepy factors," "decreased motivation" and "projection of fatigue feelings into the body." This theoretical perspective does not explain anything about the cause of the phenomenon. Nociceptors might be cancer specific;

perception and expression might be dependent on personality, history and supporting network. Results of the interviews led the researcher to build subgroups of items that take account of different expressions of fatigue at physical, affective and cognitive levels. These different levels could also be called different facets of the construct under study. Fatigue/tiredness here showed different facets, and it seemed important to differentiate between different facets of tiredness and different other constructs. It had to be kept in mind that all items should measure the same latent variable (De Vellis 1991).

Step 4: Comparison of Items Identified with Items in the Literature Reviewed

The items of the subscale "vigor/fatigue" on the POMS (McNair and Lorr 1971) include the themes worn-out, fatigued, exhausted, which were also identified in the interviews. The EORTC quality of life questionnaire subscale on fatigue (Hürny and Bernhard 1993) includes the items weakness, physical unwellness, tiredness, need for rest, as also identified in the interviews. The Piper Fatigue Scale (Piper 1992) includes some of the identified items, but mainly measures consequences of fatigue, which is not the primary target for further planned studies. The same is true in the case of the other quality of life questionnaires and ability or performance indexes reviewed; apart from the item "felt low in energy or no energy," which was also identified in the interviews, no further description of fatigue itself was identified. The scale described by Kobashi and Hanewald (1985) includes the themes tiredness, activity, illness and wellness. The Pearson-Byars Fatigue Checklist (Pearson and Byars 1956) only has one item in common with the descriptions in the interviews, which is "extremely tired"; the others, ranging from the continuum "bursting with energy" to the one "ready to drop/dead tired" seem different in nature from those identified by cancer patients. The Yoshitake Symptoms of Fatigue Checklist (Yoshitake 1971) also assesses several symptoms concerning difficulties with concentration (heavy head, difficulty in thinking and concentrating, difficulty in paying attention) and affective expressions (anxiety, impatience), and also the illness feeling, which have also been identified in the interviews.

The symptom distress scales reviewed merely used the anchor words "not tired at all" and "exhausted or could not feel more tired." In contrast, the patients in the previously described interview study frequently reported extreme, unusual tiredness.

Step 5: Identification of New Items from the Interview Study

Comparison of items in the literature reviewed and items identified in the interview study (previous chapter) showed partial correspondence. The remaining items/themes from the interviews, which were not found verbatim in the other instruments, were decreased physical performance, sleepiness in the daytime, need to force oneself to overcome inactivity, unusual need for sleep, becoming slower, wishing to switch off thoughts, sadness, wishing to withdraw, and sleeping problems at night. The item pleasant tiredness after a hard day's work or after physical exercise, which was identified in the interview study with healthy individuals, was also not found in other instruments.

Step 6: Questionnaire Design

Determining the Method and Justifying Self-Assessment

Owing to the subjectivity of fatigue, a self-reporting measurement approach was selected. Precisely because of this subjective nature of symptom distress, assessment by the patients themselves is regarded as the "gold standard" (Bruera 1991). Distress is perceived as subjective reality by the patients and has to be an accepted fact for caregivers. Fatigue measurement has similarities with pain assessment, where respect for the statement, "pain is whatever the patient says it is, whenever he says it is" (McCafferey 1979), has been described as a prerequisite for treatment. Measurement of fatigue is subjective and therefore needs to be assessed by the patients themselves. Doctors and nurses can only suspect the intensity of fatigue or observe signs or symptoms, which might be expressions of or responses to fatigue.

Determining the Multiple Dimensions

The interviews revealed that tiredness/fatigue was experienced in more than one dimension (previous chapter). Multidimensionality requires measurement from the viewpoint of its distress or negative impact on quality of life (Calmann 1987). This criterion was taken account of by the integration of questions concerning the dimensions of physical, affective and cognitive fatigue. Two additional linear analogue scales were constructed to explore the dimensions of quantity of fatigue and its severity (distress). The anchor words for the tiredness scale were "I do not feel unusually tired" and "I feel completely exhausted." This definition of the continuum was developed from the words expressed in the interviews with cancer patients and makes a clear distinction between tiredness as a normal life experience and tiredness as an unusual experience.

Determining the Response Categories and the Format for Measurement

The selection of the response categories arose from the aim of discriminating differences in the underlying attribute. As the instrument had to be easy to fill out and as protection from unnecessary burden had to be considered, the dichotomous "yes/no" format was used. This format allows nonambiguous answers and forces the respondent to make a clear decision. Concerning the tiredness items of the questionnaire, it was intended to receive a clear indication of whether the different items were part of the construct of fatigue, which would be favored by the yes/no answer. Even though variability is a desirable quality of a measurement scale (De Vellis 1991), variability concerning each item was not given highest priority in this case. Variability was expected to be measured by summing up the items in future tests.

To allow the scales included to measure unusual tiredness and the distress it causes, the format of the visual analogue scale (VAS) was chosen. High variability was necessary for sensitive quantification. Even though the interpretation of physical space, as it relates to values of the continuum, might be very subjective, VAS have been considered very helpful in the measurement of quality of life (Bindemann 1987). As tiredness is a very subjective phenomenon, it seemed that only a very sensitive measurement tool would be adequate.

Subject burden and feasibility had to be carefully considered, because the investigation had to be carried out in a vulnerable, possibly tired population. To be acceptable to ill persons, fatigue assessment tools must be short and easy to fill out. Ways of reducing subject burden and research-induced fatigue must be considered (Piper 1993). However, if a tool measures a composite of distinct factors, a distinction in correlation data must emerge; if not it could be argued that the instrument is little more than an elaborate way of asking "how do you feel?" Low subject burden is provided by the use of the single-item approach, which is a critical issue when attentional fatigue may be present (Winningham and Nail 1994). This is especially true if repeated measurement is needed. Tools need to be simple and effective, but not expensive, time-consuming or exhausting for debilitated patients. Questionnaire length is therefore a critical aspect, and redundancy of overlapping themes must be considered. Feasibility also concerns the reading level, and easy understanding of the instrument by persons with a considerable range of educational backgrounds seems crucial.

Selection of the Time Span

The questions concerned three time frames: today, last week and last month. Various time spans have been reported in the literature reviewed, ranging from right now, through today, yesterday, last week, and last fortnight to last month. During chemotherapy, a distressing symptom might occur in the first days of administration, whereas in a period of rest during which a patient recovers from short-term effects things might be different. Which period should be reported: the rest period or the treatment period - or both (Van Dam 1984)? It has been suggested that a theoretical justification for limiting the time span can be based on the distinction between state measures (how people feel or react at a particular moment, with a prescribed time frame) and trait measures (how people feel or react in general, without a time frame). The essence of a trait measure is stability over time, while state measures are expected to fluctuate with conditions that affect the relevant construct under investigation (Huismann 1987). Shorter time frames are recommended in the use of assessment of treatment-related toxicity at a particular moment, in order to minimize potential confounding by the trait disposition of the individual. Current literature reveals that the issue of time span has received relatively little attention. For the purpose of this study, the time frames today, last week and last month were selected. This decision takes into account that there might be changes over short time periods, such as tiredness caused by chemotherapy, but there might also be tiredness attributable to tumor activity over longer periods of time. It also takes into account that memory effects play a part: it seems easier to remember today or yesterday than last month. Conversely, experience shows that tiredness can become a chronic state, which could have similarities with aspects of trait, such as stability over time.

Outcome: The Fatigue Assessment Questionnaire (FAQ, Preliminary Version)

At this stage, a list of 22 questions, developed from the 22 items selected from the interviews, was generated. Ordering of the questions followed, according to the frequency with which items had been mentioned by the interviewees. The closed-ended, yes/no questions were constructed in such a way as to be easily answerable by self-assessment. Wording was carefully monitored for clarity, sensitivity, brevity, freedom from bias (for example, including more than one idea) and reading level. Questions were related to the three time frames, today, last week, and last month, so that each question would receive three answers indicated by circles round "yes" or "no." In addition, tiredness was assessed quantitatively with linear analogue scales (Linear Analogue Scale Assessment; LASA) for the time frames today, last week, and last month and one further LASA was used to assess whether this tiredness was perceived as distress during the time being measured. This distress resulting from tiredness was considered to be a global assessment of the severity of the impact of fatigue. The questions and the LASA for measurement of unusual tiredness were accompanied by short, written instructions on how to use them.

Further ongoing research can only be successful with reliability- and validity-tested instruments. Results of such a validation study would guide further development of the instruments, allow adaptations, and help to improve validity and reliability. Unbiased measurement could then offer a key to the development of therapeutic nursing and medical or psychological support measures.

At this stage, the FAQ was ready to be analyzed and tested in a validation study. It was planned that it should be used in cancer patients and in healthy individuals. Among the healthy individuals, medical research experts were to be involved in order to test the use of the questionnaire and to comment on it. These steps are described in the next chapter.

References

Aaronson K, Ahmedzai S (1993) The European Organisation for Research and Treatment of Cancer QLQ-C30: a quality of life instrument for use in international clinical trials in oncology. J Natl Cancer Inst 85 (5):365–376
Bindemann S (1987) Psychological impact of cancer: its assessment, treatment and ensuing effects on quality of life. In: Aaronson N, Beckmann J (eds) The quality of life in cancer patients. Raven Press, New York, p 227
Blesch K, Paice J (1991) Correlates of fatigue in breast or lung cancer. Oncol Nurs Forum 18:81–87
Bruera E (1991) The Edmonton Symptom Assessment System (ESAS): a simple method for the assessment of palliative care patients. J Palliat Care 7 (2):6–9
Cahmann K (1987) Definition and dimensions of quality of life. In: Aaronson N, Beckmann J (eds) The quality of life in cancer patients. Raven Press, New York, p 1
CARES Consultants (1988) Cancer Rehabilitation Evaluation System. Oncology 4 (5):212
Cella D (1990) Functional assessment of cancer therapy (FACT).Oncology 4 (5):216 [Appendix]
Cella D, Orofiamma B (1987) The relationship between psychological distress, extent of disease, and performance status in patients with lung cancer. Cancer 60:1661–1667
Cronbach L (1951) Coefficient alpha and the internal structure of tests. Psychometrika 16 (3):297–335
De Vellis R (1991) Scale development. Sage, Newbury Park
Field P, Morse J (1985) Nursing research. The application of qualitative approaches. Chapman and Hall, London
Fox B (1995) Some problems and some solutions in research on psychotherapeutic intervention in cancer. Support Care Cancer 3:257–263
Freel M, Hart L (1977) Study of fatigue phenomena of multiple sclerosis patients (USDEW Grant no 5R02-NU-00534-02). University of Iowa, Division of Nursing, Iowa City
Glaus A (1993) Assessment of fatigue in cancer and non-cancer patients and in healthy individuals. Support Care Cancer 1:305–315
Haylock P, Hart L (1979) Fatigue in patients receiving localised radiation. Cancer Nurs 2:461–467
Heinrich R, Schag C (1983) Psychosocial problem specification with cancer patients. Clin Res 31:408 (abstract)
Holmes S (1991) Preliminary investigation of symptom distress in two cancer patient populations: evaluation of a measurement instrument. J Adv Nurs 16:439–446
Huismann S, van Dam F (1987) On measuring complaints of cancer patients: some remarks on the time span question. In: Aaronson N, Beckmann J (eds) The quality of life in cancer patients. Raven Press, New York, p 101
Hürny C, Bernhard J (1993) "Fatigue and malaise" as a quality of life indicator in small-cell lung cancer patients. The Swiss Group for Clinical Cancer Research. Support Care Cancer 1:316–320
Izak F, Medalie J (1971) Comprehensive follow-up of carcinoma patients. J Chron Dis 24:179–191
Jamar S (1989) Fatigue in women receiving chemotherapy for ovarian cancer. In: Funk, S, Tornquist M (eds) Key aspects of comfort: management of pain, fatigue and nausea. Springer, Berlin Heidelberg New York, pp 224–233
Karnofsky D, Abelmann W (1948) The use of the nitrogen mustards in the palliative treatment of carcinoma. Cancer 1:634–656
Kobashi J, Hanewald G (1985) Assessment of malaise in cancer patients treated with radiotherapy. Cancer Nurs 12:306–313
Levin M, Guyatt G (1988) Quality of life in stage II breast cancer: an instrument for clinical trials. J Clin Oncol 6 (12):1798–1810
McCafferey M (1979) Nursing management of the patient in pain, 2nd edn. Lippincott, Philadelphia, p 32

McCorkle R, Young K (1978) Development of a symptom distress scale. Cancer Nurs 10:373–378
McNair D, Lorr M (1971) EITS manual for the profile of mood states. Educational and Industrial Testing Service, San Diego
Nunnally J (1978) Psychometric theory, 2nd edn. McGraw Hill, New York
Padilla G, Presant C (1983) Quality of life index for patients with cancer. Res Nurs Health 6:117–126
Pearson P, Byars G (1956) The development and validation of a checklist measuring subjective fatigue (report no. 56–115). School of Aviation, Randolph AFB, TX
Piper B (1992) Subjective fatigue in women receiving six cycles of adjuvant chemotherapy for breast cancer. PhD dissertation, University of California, San Francisco. Ann Arbor, MI: UMI dissertation services (no 9303553)
Piper B (1993) Fatigue. In: Carrieri V, Lindsey A (eds) Pathophysiological phenomena in nursing: human response to illness. Saunders, Philadelphia
Piper B, Lindsey A (1987) Fatigue mechanisms in cancer patients: developing nursing theory. Oncol Nurs Forum 14:17–23
Piper B, Lindsey A (1989) The development of an instrument to measure the subjective dimension of fatigue. In: Funk S, Tornquist A (1989) Key aspects of comfort. Springer, Berlin Heidelberg New York
Polit D, Hungler B (1993) Nursing research, principles and methods. Lippincott, Philadelphia
Rhoten D (1982) Fatigue in the postsurgical patient. In: Norris C (ed) concept clarification in nursing. Aspen, Rockville, pp 277–300
Schag C, Heinrich R (1984) Karnofsky performance status revisited: reliability, validity and guidelines. J Clin Oncol 2 (3):187–193
Schipper H, Clinch J (1984) Measuring the quality of life of cancer patients: the Functional Living Index-Cancer: development and validation. J Clin Oncol 2 (5):123–136
Smith N (1993) Quality of life studies from the perspective of an FDA reviewing statistician. Drug Inform J 27:617–623
Van Dam F, Linssen A (1984) Evaluating quality of life: behavioural measures in clinical trials. In: Buyse M, Staquet M (eds) Cancer clinical trials: methods and practice. Oxford University Press, New York, p 98
Winningham M, Nail M (1994) Fatigue and the cancer experience: the state of the knowledge. Oncol Nurs Forum 21 (1):23–36
World Health Organisation (1990) Cancer pain relief and palliative care. WHO, Geneva (WHO technical report series 804)
Yoshitake H (1971) Relations between the symptoms and feelings of fatigue. Ergonomics 14:175–186
Zubrod C, Schneidermann M (1960) Appraisal of methods for the study of chemotherapy of cancer in man: comparative therapeutic trial of nitrogen mustard and triethylene thiophosphoramide. J Chron Dis 11:7–33

Testing the Fatigue Assessment Questionnaire in Healthy Persons and in Cancer Patients

Introduction

In the past decade, measurement of fatigue has become an important quality of life issue, especially in the field of nursing (Winningham and Nail 1994). Lack of clarification of the concept has led to difficulties in its measurement. Studies about prevalence, correlates and possible causes are difficult to compare owing to methodological differences (Piper 1993). A review of currently available fatigue measurement instruments has led to the conclusion that for the purpose of epidemiological research with the aim of measuring the experience of fatigue in a general cancer patient population, no valid instrument is available. Previously conducted, unstructured interviews with cancer patients and healthy individuals (above) therefore formed the basis of the analysis of the descriptors of fatigue from the perspective of those concerned. These descriptors were compared with items in available instruments and then used to construct a self-report Fatigue Assessment Questionnaire (FAQ). Construction of this scale has been described in the last chapter. As only research conducted with reliability- and validity-tested instruments can be successful, the FAQ now needs to be scientifically tested.

Aim of the Study

It was the aim of this study to test the new Fatigue Assessment Questionnaire (FAQ) with reference to reliability and validity, feasibility and acceptability and, further, to generate knowledge concerning the concept of fatigue in cancer patients.

Study Design, Setting, Population, and Selection

A nonrandomized, explorative, prospective design was used to test the fatigue questionnaire in healthy individuals and in cancer patients. The inclusion of a subpopulation of healthy individuals means the design could be described as quasi-experimental, as they served as a baseline subpopulation allowing a distinction between healthy and diseased individuals. With a cross-sectional design, the phenomena under investigation were captured as they manifested themselves at the period of data collection and were related to external variables. A descriptive and correlational approach was used to portray the characteristics and to investigate any interrelationships among variables of interest.

Study Setting and Population

The study was conducted in the Department of Internal Medicine C (Oncology, Hematology, Gastroenterology) of the Kantonsspital St. Gallen, Switzerland, a 900-bed teaching hospital. Subject accrual took place from March to June 1995.

The study population was made up of two subpopulations:

1 Seventy-seven (77) healthy individuals, working in the hospital setting as nurses, doctors, technicians, secretaries, volunteers
2 Seventy-seven (77) consecutive cancer patients, who came to the hospital for treatment and care

Selection/Entry Criteria

The healthy subpopulation was selected according to availability in the environment of the researcher in the hospital. The criterion for classification as healthy was the ability to perform fully and as usual in the job setting and in the personal environment, without disease-induced limitation. To assure representativeness of the healthy subpopulation and to fulfill the criteria of homogeneity, age and gender were controlled. Subjects also had to be able to understand and read the German language.

The subpopulation of cancer patients was selected according to their availability in the department. For the period of accrual, every incoming inpatient with known neoplasm was considered for investigation, if possible within the first three days of admission, so that changes resulting from further treatment or deterioration could be ascertained. In the outpatient department, different subjects were selected on each week day (Monday to Friday), in order to avoid selection bias, which could otherwise have resulted from selection of specific patient groups scheduled for specific days. Representativeness of this sample was given, as it was drawn from a general cancer patient population.

Criteria for exclusion from the study were: not yet histologically confirmed neoplasm, cognitive impairment, known brain metastasis, psychiatric disorders, not understanding/reading the German language.

Methods

Instruments

The Fatigue Assessment Questionnaire

The FAQ for self-assessment (German version) was used to assess expression, quantity and distress of fatigue within the time spans "today," "last week," and "last month." This new questionnaire measures the physical, affective and cognitive expression of fatigue with 22 items and quantity and distress of fatigue with linear analogue scales. As the purpose of the FAQ was epidemiological fatigue research, items had dichotomous answers (yes/no), which was expected to result in clear-cut decisions by the patients.

The Hospital Anxiety and Depression Scale

HADS, the Hospital Anxiety and Depression scale, was used at the same time to assess the items within the time span of last week. This scale was originally developed to detect anxiety and depression in medical patients. Concepts of emotional and physical illness are separated, and evidence was presented that the scale scores were not affected by the presence of physical illness (Zigmond and Snaith 1983). The scale has been translated into the German language, and reliability and validity have been established with success (Herrmann and Scholz 1991). The scale includes seven items concerning depression and seven items concerning anxiety. This instrument was chosen because of its ability to distinguish between emotional and physical symptoms, which is especially important in a population with cancer. The aim was to detect anxiety and depression as separate concepts in relation to tiredness and to assess their correlational occurrence.

The Karnofsky Index

For the subpopulation of cancer patients, the Karnofsky Index was assessed by the investigator. This numerical scale from 0 to 100 represents the patients' ability to perform normal activity, the ability to do active work, and the need for assistance in activities of daily living (Karnofsky and Burchenal 1949). It has been widely tested and used for making clinical decisions in the treatment of cancer (Schag and Heinrich 1984). This index was expected to show correlations between activity status and tiredness.

Patient Characteristics: Sociodemographic, Health-Related and Medical Data

Patients and healthy individuals were asked to fill out a questionnaire concerning sociodemographic and health-related data: date and place of investigation, initials, age, gender, profession, ability to work, marital status, regular intake of medications. Concerning health status, subjects responded to the question as to whether they (1) were healthy, (2) were healthy but suffering from an acute disturbance (e.g., influenza), or (3) suffered from a chronic disease and, if this was the case, which disease.

For the subpopulation of cancer patients, additional, medical data were collected by the investigator: type of tumor, stage of disease, tumor activity, treatment and kind of treatment at the time of the investigation and within the last 6 weeks (none, chemotherapy, hormonal treatment, immune therapy, radiotherapy, surgery), other medications and in- or outpatient status. These data were expected to be useful for detection of correlations between tiredness and external variables in cancer patients.

Procedures

Before the start of data collection, the investigator had to train the research assistant in administration of the self-assessment instruments (how to fill out, sequence of administration, time frames required) and how to use the Karnofsky scale, which revealed the need for guidelines, as had been described by Schag and Heinrich (1984). Careful briefing was expected to avoid introduction of bias.

The first five patients served as pilot users to test the comprehensibility of the new questionnaire and to assess the feasibility of the instruments in this population. Slight adaptations had to be made. This was also the case for the forms concerning sociodemographic data and medical data collection, and especially for questions of coding and the translation of data into categories of numeric form to ensure easy transfer from written documents to computer files for statistical analysis.

Questionnaires were coded with numbers to provide for confidentiality. The first 20 questionnaires were sent to healthy individuals, all of them leading physicians, most of them involved in research. They were not only asked to fill out the instruments, but were invited to share their experience of the questionnaire and to comment on it. The purpose of this was to gain access to a judgment on the structure and comprehensibility of the tiredness questionnaire from the viewpoint of users as scientists. Three of them each wrote a helpful comment (two drawing attention to the use of two adjectives in a question; one questioning the meaning of words). The other healthy subjects were approached individually, apart from a group of nurses (20 nurses), who were instructed in a group session.

Cancer patients were approached individually in the outpatient department or at the bedside by the researcher, according to the selection criteria. They were first asked for their willingness to participate and to give oral consent. Patients were assured confidentiality in the sense that only the researcher would have access to the data and be able to identify the person. The purpose of the inquiry was then explained, and instructions were given on how to fill out the questionnaire and in what order (first the fatigue questionnaire, then the HAD Scale, followed by the demographic data sheet).

This order of the instruments was chosen because it was thought that providing the sociodemographic data might demotivate people who were otherwise willing to take part in the inquiry. Most of the patients were then left alone to complete the instruments, which were picked up later. On this occasion, open questions could be answered and the questionnaire was screened for missing data and the patients asked whether these had been left out on purpose. This method of data collection is said to ensure a high response rate, accurate sampling and a minimum of interviewer bias, while permitting interviewer assessments, providing necessary explanations and giving the benefit of a degree of personal contact (Oppenheim 1992).

Statistical Analysis

Data were transferred from written documents to a data base (Filemaker). Statistical analyses were performed with the statistical program SAS, with the exception of the Cronbach alpha correlation coefficients, which were calculated with STATA 3.2. Descriptive statistics were used to classify data and to give information about the characteristics of the study population. For statistical analysis, the dichotomous answers in the tiredness questionnaire first required coding. Fisher's two-tailed exact test was used to test differences in proportions in 2×2 contingency tables formed by cross tabulation of items from the questionnaire with health status (healthy persons versus cancer patients, univariate discrimination). The phi correlation coefficient (preferred for dichotomous variables) was used to examine the magnitude of the association of health status with the items of the questionnaire for the three different time spans of their measurement (Polit and Hungler 1993).

Logistic regression (preferred if nominal measurement is involved) was used to analyze the relationship between items (multivariate discrimination) and health status and to determine redundant items. Logistic regression is a method used to predict or explain the values of one variable in terms of the remaining variables (Nigel 1993). *p*-values for the results of logistic regression were calculated using the Wald chi-square test.

Construct validity of the instrument was examined by factor analysis (results from varimax rotation, promax rotation and procrustes rotation). Construct validation is aimed at ascertaining whether the relation between the variables measured is consistent with prior expectations on the basis of an underlying theory of the aspects investigated (Jones et al. 1987). Factor analysis is used to disentangle complex interrelationships among variables and identifies which variables go together as unified concepts or factors. It is described as a method for examining dimensions of complex characteristics and used as an heuristic, hypothesis-generating technique (Bortz 1985). Internal consistency of the tiredness questionnaire was examined using Cronbach alpha correlation coefficients.

The Wilcoxon test (instead of a *t* test, because of skewed data) was used to test for differences between healthy and diseased individuals in median scores for fatigue and fatigue-related distress and median scores on the HAD Scales. The Pearson correlation coefficient was used for the correlation between intensity of tiredness and the distress arising from it, as measured by the Karnofsky Index (interval scale) and the HAD scales (ordinal scales). To examine criterion-related validity, tiredness was compared between healthy and diseased individuals with the Wilcoxon test. Differences in proportions concerning items of the HAD scales in healthy and diseased individuals were tested with the chi-square test and estimated with phi coefficients, and differences of location were assessed with the Wilcoxon test. Content validity was supported by the fact that the questionnaire items had been collected in open-ended interviews with cancer patients and healthy individuals and that these interviews had been content-analyzed according to a grounded theory approach until data saturation was achieved (Field and Morse 1985).

Ethical Approval/Patient Consent

The study was approved by the ethical committee of the Kantonsspital and by the medical and nursing director of the department. Patients and healthy individuals were asked for oral consent to be involved in the study. Confidentiality was respected by coding of the questionnaires.

Results

Characteristics of the Populations

Healthy Individuals

One hundred five (105) healthy individuals were asked to participate in the study: 19 did not send back the questionnaire and 86 were returned, which represents a response rate of 82%. The 86 returned included 9 that were not eligible, for the following reasons: empty questionnaire returned (4), no health-related information given (2), cancer (1), missing data (2). Eventually, 77 healthy individuals were eligible for the study, which represents eligibility of data in 90%.

Table 1 presents the characteristics of the subpopulation of healthy individuals. Females and males were equally distributed. Fifty-six percent of the healthy individuals were women and 44% percent, men. Mean age was 54 years (standard deviation 12.82, range 18–76). Of the 77 healthy individuals, 8 suffered from a chronic health disturbance other than cancer. All 77 subjects in this subsample considered themselves to be in a healthy condition. Assessment of medication intake revealed that few individuals used psychotropic drugs (3%), sleep medication (1%), or pain medication (1%), but 23% of this subpopulation did use some other type of medication.

Table 1. Characteristics of the study populations

		Cancer patients ($n=77$)	Healthy persons ($n=77$)
Gender	Female	48%	56%
	Male	52%	44%
Age (years)	Mean	53[a]	54[b]
	Range	17–78	18–76
Medications (other than cancer drugs)			23%
Karnofsky Index	100	30%	
	80–90	56%	
	Below 80	14%	
Diagnosis	Lung cancer	12%	
	Breast cancer	16%	
	Lymphomas/leukemia	30%	
	Gastrointestinal cancer	19%	
	Other tumors	23%	
Disease state	Distant metastasis	75%	
	Regional metastasis	14%	
	Disease free	11%	
Treatment	Chemotherapy	81%	
	Hormone therapy	9%	
	Immune therapy	5%	
	Radiotherapy	8%	
	Surgery	1%	
Status	Inpatient	43%	
	Outpatient	57%	

[a] SD = 15.77.
[b] SD = 12.82.

Cancer Patients

In all, 98 cancer patients were asked to participate in the study; 9 of them declined and 3 did not return the questionnaire, which represents a response rate of 87%. There were 9 patients who did not qualify [language problems (3), worsening condition (4), unclear diagnosis (1), cognitive inability (1)]. Seventy-seven cancer patients were finally eligible, which represents eligibility of data in 88% of the subpopulation.

Table 1 also presents the characteristics of the cancer patients. Female and male gender were almost equally represented, with 48% female and 52% male patients. Mean age was 53 years (standard deviation 15.77, range 17–78). Cancer diagnoses were classified into lung cancer, breast cancer, lymphomas/leukemia, gastrointestinal cancers and other solid tumors. The Karnofsky Index was 100 in 30% of the patients, 80–90 in 56%, and below 80 in

14%. Most (75%) were suffering from systemic disease and 14% from regional disease; 11% had no evidence of tumor. Fifteen of the 77 patients (19%) had no treatment. The remaining 81% were receiving cancer treatment, including chemotherapy, hormone treatment, immune therapy and radiotherapy, at the time of investigation, and only 1% had surgery within the last 6 weeks. Fifty-seven percent of the cancer patient subpopulation were treated as outpatients and 43% were admitted for inpatient care.

Individuals needed approximately 15 min to complete the study forms. Most managed independently, only a few patients needing some assistance.

Univariate Discrimination of the Questionnaire Items

Discriminating Between the Two Subpopulations in Three Time Spans

The 22 items of the tiredness questionnaire were examined according to the three time spans "today," "last week," and "last month" and were statistically analyzed using Fisher's two-tailed exact test, to discriminate responses from healthy individuals from those of cancer patients. The results are presented in Table 2 (see pp. 86, 87). For the time span today highly significant differences ($p \leq 0.01$) were found between healthy persons and cancer patients for the items decreased physical performance, unusual, extreme tiredness, weakness, sleepiness in the daytime, unusual need for rest, fight to overcome inactivity, becoming slower, and loss of energy, loss of interest and general unwellness. Weak significance ($p \leq 0.05$) was found for the items pleasant tiredness, heavy limbs, impaired attentiveness, unusual need for sleep, wish to switch off thoughts, sleeping disorders. No significant difference ($p \geq 0.05$) was found for the items exhaustion, impaired concentration, sadness, feeling impatient, anxiety, and wish to withdraw.

Between the time span "today" and the time span "last week" only two of the weakly significant items change: pleasant tiredness and sleeping disorders become significant for last week (from weakly significant for today). The items anxiety and impaired concentration became weakly significant ($p \leq 0.05$) for last week but were not significant for today. The items heavy limbs, impaired attentiveness and wish to switch off thoughts became nonsignificant for last week but were weakly significant ($p \leq 0.05$) for "today." Four further items remained nonsignificant for the time span "last week."

Only one of the significantly different items changed from last week to last month: anxiety increased in significance for last month. The item sleeping disorders was weakly significant for last week but not significant for last month. The items impaired concentration and sleeping disorders lost significance for the period of last month in comparison with last week, as they were for the time span today.

Items With No Change Over the Three Time Spans

Decreased physical performance, unusual tiredness, weakness, sleepiness in the daytime, unusual need for rest, need to fight to overcome inactivity, becoming slower, loss of energy and general unwellness remained highly significantly different between healthy and diseased individuals through all three time spans ($p \leq 0.01$). Significance was found in all three time spans for unusual need for sleep ($p \leq 0.05$). No difference between healthy and diseased individuals was found in any of the three time spans for the items exhaustion, sadness, feeling impatient and wish to withdraw ($p \geq 0.05$).

Magnitude of Association Between Health Status and Questionnaire Items

Examination of the magnitude of the association between health status and the items of the questionnaire for the three time spans revealed rather modest phi coefficients (Table 2). Moderately high coefficients (>0.40) were found for association with the items decreased physical performance, weakness, fight to overcome inactivity, becoming slow and loss of energy. Moderately low (<0.20) were the coefficients of association with the items pleasant tiredness (minus values), exhaustion, heavy limbs, attentiveness, concentration, sadness, feeling impatient, anxiety, and wish to withdraw.

Logistic Regression of the Questionnaire Items in the Two Subpopulations in Three Time Spans

Logistic regression was carried out to analyze the relationship between the items and to detect redundant items. Results are presented in Table 3. From the 22 items, 11 remained significantly different between healthy and diseased individuals at a significance level of 0.20 for the time span of today, 10 for the time span of last week, and 12 for the time span of last month. The items pleasant tiredness, decreased physical performance, weakness, fight to overcome inactivity and becoming slower remained significant over all three time spans. The items unusual, extreme tiredness, unusual need for rest, impaired concentration, unusual need for sleep, wish to switch off thoughts and general unwellness showed no significant discrimination from other items, remaining nonsignificant over all three time spans. Owing to their conceptual importance, these items were retained for further analysis. As the item "wish to switch off thoughts" had shown only a weak difference for today in the univariate analysis and now showed no difference in the multivariate analysis, it was considered to be deleted for further analysis.

Investigation of the Three Time Spans Measured in the 77 Cancer Patients

In the sample with cancer patients, the phi coefficient was calculated for all questionnaire items and cross-correlations of the time spans today/last week,

Table 2. Univariate discrimination of items in the Fatigue Assessment Questionnaire (n=77 healthy individuals and 77 cancer patients)

	Time span					
	Today		Last week		Last month	
	p	Phi coefficient	p	Phi coefficient	p	Phi coefficient
Fatigue/tiredness item						
1 Pleasant tiredness	0.037*	−0.17	0.001**	−0.27	≤0.001**	0.29
2 Decreased physical performance	≤0.001**	0.51	≤0.001**	0.52	≤0.001**	0.45
3 Unusual, extreme tiredness	≤0.001**	0.30	≤0.001**	0.30	0.001**	0.28
4 Exhaustion/feel worn out	0.347	0.08	0.420	0.08	0.051	0.17
5 Heavy limbs	0.016*	0.20	0.54	0.08	0.299	0.09
6 Weakness	≤0.001**	0.40	≤0.001**	0.47	≤0.001**	0.44
7 Sleepiness in daytime	0.001**	0.27	0.001**	0.27	≤0.001**	0.34
8 Unusual need for rest	≤0.001**	0.35	≤0.001** 0.36	≤0.001**	0.31	
9 Fight to overcome inactivity	≤0.001**	0.43	≤0.001**	0.42	≤0.001**	0.45
10 Impaired concentration	0.131	0.14	0.014*	0.21	0.054	0.16
11 Impaired attentiveness	0.028*	0.19	0.086	0.15	0.210	0.12
12 Sadness	0.157	0.13	0.106	0.14	0.097	0.15
13 Feeling impatient	0.588	0.07	0.079	−0.16	0.091	−0.15
14 Unusual need for sleep	0.017*	0.20	0.015*	0.21	0.014*	0.31
15 Becoming slower	≤0.001**	0.40	≤0.001**	0.37	≤0.001**	0.38

Table 2 (Continued)

16 Wish to switch off thoughts	0.014*	0.24	0.083	0.15	0.231	0.11
17 Anxiety	0.100	0.15	0.012*	0.21	0.003**	0.24
18 Loss of energy	≤0.001**	0.56	≤0.001**	0.47	≤0.001**	0.48
19 Loss of interest	0.004**	0.23	0.036*	0.17	0.017*	0.20
20 Wish to withdraw	0.442	0.07	0.498	0.06	0.618	–0.05
21 Sleep disorders	0.020*	0.20	0.003**	0.24	0.134	0.13
22 General unwellness	0.001**	0.27	0.007**	0.23	0.001**	0.26

Fisher's exact test, two tailed.
$*p \leq 0.05$; $** \ p \leq 0.01$.

Table 3. Logistic regression analysis of items in the Fatigue Assessment Questionnaire ($n=77$ healthy individuals and 77 cancer patients)

	Time span		
	Today *p*	Last week *p*	Last month *p*
Fatigue/tiredness item			
1 Pleasant tiredness	0.01	0.01	0.04
2 Decreased physical performance	0.01	0.02	0.04
3 Unusual, extreme tiredness	*	*	*
4 Exhaustion/feel worn out	0.01	0.12	*
5 Heavy limbs	*	0.02	0.02
6 Weakness	0.19	0.06	0.09
7 Sleepiness in daytime	0.20	0.05	*
8 Unusual need for rest	*	*	*
9 Fight to overcome inactivity	0.03	0.06	0.05
10 Impaired concentration	*	*	*
11 Impaired attentiveness	*	*	0.20
12 Sadness	0.16	*	0.07
13 Feeling impatient	*	0.03	0.04
14 Unusual need for sleep	*	*	*
15 Becoming slower	0.06	0.14	0.02
16 Wish to switch off thoughts	*	*	*
17 Anxiety	*	*	0.07
18 Loss of energy	0.06	*	0.15
19 Loss of interest	0.15	*	*
20 Wish to withdraw	0.10	*	0.07
21 Sleep disorders	*	0.02	*
22 General unwellness	*	*	*

Wald chi-square test.
p at 0.20 level (partial *p* value); *, no discrimination.

today/last month, last week/last month were calculated to examine the influence of the time frame on items. Results are presented in Table 4. Cross-correlation between today and last week showed that 16 items had correlations between 0.70 and 0.96, with loss of interest and becoming slower being ranked highest. Five items, exhaustion, feel impatient, anxiety, loss of energy and wish to withdraw, showed correlation coefficients between 0.50 and 0.69 and only 1 item, sadness (0.33), had a value under 0.50. Cross-correlation between today and last month showed only the 5 items, heavy limbs, weakness, becoming slower, wish to switch off thoughts, and loss of interest, with a cor-

Table 4. Cross correlation of items related to three time spans in 77 cancer patients (Phi coefficients)

	Time spans correlated		
	Today/last week	Today/last month	Last week/last month
Fatigue/tiredness item			
1 Pleasant tiredness	0.71	0.55	0.76
2 Decreased physical performance	0.73	0.66	0.78
3 Unusual, extreme tiredness	0.84	0.67	0.76
4 Exhaustion/feel worn out	0.61	0.49	0.60
5 Heavy limbs	0.87	0.73	0.83
6 Weakness	0.83	0.70	0.85
7 Sleepiness in daytime	0.72	0.60	0.72
8 Unusual need for rest	0.77	0.63	0.69
9 Fight to overcome inactivity	0.72	0.56	0.72
10 Impaired concentration	0.74	0.55	0.68
11 Impaired attentiveness	0.71	0.64	0.73
12 Sadness	0.48	0.33	0.56
13 Feeling impatient	0.51	0.45	0.54
14 Unusual need for sleep	0.70	0.45	0.69
15 Becoming slower	0.92	0.74	0.82
16 Wish to switch off thoughts	0.78	0.72	0.83
17 Anxiety	0.50	0.41	0.67
18 Loss of energy	0.68	0.53	0.73
19 Loss of interest	0.96	0.77	0.81
20 Wish to withdraw	0.64	0.50	0.61
21 Sleep disorders	0.71	0.50	0.68
22 General unwellness	0.70	0.56	0.55

relation coefficient between 0.70 and 0.77, while for 12 items they were between 0.50 and 0.69 and for 5 items, exhaustion, sadness, feeling impatient, unusual need for sleep and anxiety, under 0.50. For the cross-correlation between last week and last month, 12 items showed a correlation between 0.70 and 0.85 and 10 items, one between 0.50 and 0.69; no item had a correlation coefficient under 0.50.

Factor Analysis of the Questionnaire Items

Questionnaire items were examined for their relationships among each other and for identification of unified concepts, using factor analysis followed by

Table 5. Factor analysis after varimax rotation of items in the Fatigue Assessment Questionnaire ($n=65$ cancer patients)

Tiredness items	Factor 1	Factor 2	Factor 3	Single factor=Δ
1 Pleasant tiredness	−0.01984	−0.13733	**−0.64253**	
2 Decreased physical performance	**0.66390**	0.39081	−0.05421	
3 Unusual tiredness	0.67216	0.00360	0.50542	Δ
4 Exhaustion	0.25230	0.33461	**0.55290**	
5 Heavy limbs	0.35851	0.09545	**0.66988**	
6 Weakness	**0.76343**	0.23360	0.28162	
7 Sleepiness in daytime	**0.65784**	0.26739	0.04725	
8 Unusual need for rest	**0.78340**	0.02280	0.26065	
9 Fight to overcome inactivity	**0.82560**	0.22624	0.08632	
10 Impaired concentration	0.06330	**0.74727**	0.18340	
11 Impaired attentiveness	0.15694	**0.70287**	0.23565	
12 Sadness	0.11392	**0.50737**	0.05266	
13 Feeling impatient	−0.17365	**0.62760**	0.19508	
14 Unusual need for sleep	0.55369	−0.09742	0.42436	Δ
15 Becoming slower	0.34622	0.46495	0.11704	Δ
16 Wish switch off thoughts				Deleted
17 Anxiety	0.11327	**0.44926**	−0.04549	
18 Loss of energy	0.70575	0.50830	0.06236	Δ
19 Loss of interest	**0.48796**	0.00204	0.00292	
20 Wish to withdraw	0.40440	0.50552	−0.38149	Δ
21 Sleeping disorders	0.18267	0.01546	0.04309	Δ
22 General unwellness	0.43176	0.22957	0.40672	Δ

varimax rotation. Results are presented in Table 5 (factor-related items printed in bold). Three factors and seven single-factor items were identified. Factor 1 comprised six items, presenting predominantly physical tiredness aspects such as decreased physical performance, weakness, sleepiness in the daytime, unusual need for rest, fight to overcome inactivity, and loss of interest. Factor 2 comprised five items with affective and cognitive aspects, such as impaired concentration, impaired attentiveness, sadness, feeling impatient and anxiety. Factor 3 comprised three items that reflected a different kind of physical tiredness, such as pleasant tiredness, exhaustion and heavy limbs. Seven items were not identified with any one of the three factors, even though their factor loadings were highest among factor 1, apart from becoming slower, which had higher loadings in factor 2. The item wish to switch off thoughts was deleted for the reasons described earlier.

A confirmatory factor analysis (procrustes rotation) was done additionally in search of support for the researcher's previous tentative theoretical frame-

Table 6. Researcher's concept (derived from the qualitative interviews) for the Fatigue Assessment Questionnaire, before factor analysis of the questionnaire items

Physical tiredness $r=0.82$	Cognitive tiredness $r=0.69$	Affective tiredness $r=0.69$
Decreased physical performance	Impaired concentration	Sadness
Weakness	Impaired attentiveness	Anxiety
Unusual need for rest	Becoming slower	Feeling impatient
Fight to overcome inactivity	Sleepiness in daytime	Wish to withdraw
Pleasant tiredness		Loss of energy
Exhaustion		General unwellness
Heavy limbs		Loss of interest
Unusual need for sleep		Sleeping problems at night
Unusual tiredness		

r, Cronbach alpha correlation coefficient.

Table 7. Factor analysis during development of the Fatigue Assessment Questionnaire: formation of clusters/subscales (1-week time span). For the entire scale $r=0.88$

Factor 1 $r=0.84$	Factor 2 $r=0.63$	Factor 3 $r=0.47$	Single items
Decreased physical performance	Impaired concentration	Pleasant tiredness	Unusual need for sleep
Weakness	Impaired attentiveness	Exhaustion	Becoming slower
Sleepiness in daytime	Sadness	Heavy limbs	Loss of energy
Unusual need for rest	Feeling impatient		Wish to withdraw
Fight to overcome inactivity	Anxiety		General unwellness
Loss of interest			Sleep problems
			Unusual tiredness

r, Cronbach alpha correlation coefficient.

work of tiredness. Results did not differ essentially from those obtained by varimax rotation.

Theory Development: Relating Factor Analyses to the Concept

Prior to factor analysis, the researcher had developed a theoretical framework to explain the expression of tiredness in cancer patients. The framework was made up of three types of expression, namely physical, cognitive, and affective tiredness, as had been suggested by the results from earlier described, qualitative research. This concept is presented in Tables 6 and 7. Reliability coefficients (Cronbach alpha) were calculated for the subscales of the original concept; these were 0.82 for the physical, 0.69 for the cognitive and 0.69 for the affective expression of tiredness. This framework partially complied with the items in the subscales from the factor analysis (Table 7). Items in factor 1 (r=0.84) mainly equaled physical expression related to the functional capacity of the body. The items of factor 3 (with an unsatisfactory correlation coefficient of 0.47) also represented some kind of physical tiredness, rather physical sen-

Table 8. Intensity and distress of tiredness assessed with LASA (Linear Analogue Scale Assessment) scales in healthy individuals ($n=77$) and cancer patients ($n=77$)

Time span	Healthy individuals (median, mm)	Cancer patients (median, mm)	p^a
Today	13	38	0.001
Last week	24	38	0.004
Last month	29	44	0.006
Distress of tiredness (median, mm)	28	43	0.003

[a] Wilcoxon test.

sations or feelings. Some of the items subsumed under factor 2 ($r=0.63$) could be allocated to cognitive and affective tiredness of the original concept. Single items appeared to be linked with all three levels of expression. The reliability coefficient (Cronbach alpha) for the entire scale was 0.88.

Assessment of Intensity of Tiredness/Fatigue and Resultant Distress and Their Correlation with the Karnofsky Index and HAD Scale Scores

Intensity of tiredness, as assessed with the LASA (Linear Analogue Scale Assessment) scale on tiredness, is presented in Table 8. Healthy individuals showed a consistent increase from today to last week to last month, whereas cancer patients showed equal intensity of tiredness today and last week, tending to increase for the period of last month. The difference between median intensity of tiredness in the two samples was statistically significant; however, the difference was even more pronounced for today ($p=0.001$) than for last week ($p=0.004$) and last month ($p=0.006$), as calculated with the Wilcoxon test.

The same was the case for the distress caused by tiredness. Median distress, presented in Table 8, was higher in cancer patients (43 mm) than in healthy individuals (28 mm), and this difference was significant ($p=0.003$).

The relationship of the Karnofsky Index with tiredness intensity, the distress experienced because of it, and the HAD scale was also examined. The results are presented in Table 9. Low and equal values are shown for correlation of the Karnofsky Index with intensity of and distress from tiredness. The correlation was higher with the HAD Depression scores than with the HAD Anxiety scores. The ratio of the HAD scales was higher for tiredness distress than for tiredness intensity. Relatively low correlations were found between tiredness and anxiety and depression scores.

HAD Scale Scores in the Two Study Subpopulations

The HAD scales were also examined in relation to the two samples. Results are presented in Table 10. Discrimination between healthy and diseased per-

Table 9. Correlation between tiredness intensity, tiredness distress, Hospital Anxiety and Depression (HAD) scale scores and Karnofsky Index

		Correlation (r)[a]
Karnofsky Index	Tiredness intensity (LASA)	0.24
Karnofsky Index	Tiredness distress (LASA)	0.26
Karnofsky Index	HAD-D scale	0.36
Karnofsky Index	HAD-A scale	0.11
HAD-A	Tiredness intensity	0.33
HAD-D	Tiredness intensity	0.37
HAD-A	Tiredness distress	0.48
HAD-D	Tiredness distress	0.54

[a] Pearson correlation coefficient.

Table 10. Results of HAD scale (German version) univariate discrimination between 77 cancer patients and 77 healthy individuals

Items (translated from German into English)	Phi coefficient	*p* value[a]
A1 (tension/irritation)	0.19	0.144
A2 (anxious presentiments)	0.28	0.007
A3 (worrying thoughts)	0.10	0.697
A4 (ability to relax)	0.24	0.030
A5 (anxious feeling in the stomach)	0.16	0.257
A6 (restlessness)	0.23	0.042
A7 (panic attacks)	0.17	0.116
D1 (ability to enjoy as before)	0.11	0.565
D2 (laughing and seeing funny things)	0.12	0.538
D3 (happiness)	0.19	0.144
D4 (feeling held back)	0.37	≤0.001
D5 (loss of interest in appearance)	0.15	0.155
D6 (enjoy future)	0.16	0.273
D7 (enjoying a book, radio, television)	0.09	0.771

Median for anxiety: 4 in healthy individuals ($n=76$) and 5 in cancer patients ($n=76$); Wilcoxon $p=0.27$; median for depression: 2.5 in healthy individuals ($n=74$) and 3 in cancer patients ($n=77$); Wilcoxon: $p=0.02$.
[a] Chi-square test.

sons revealed low phi coefficients for anxiety (0.16–0.28) and also for depression (0.11–0.37). Chi-square tests showed significance (≤0.01) for the anxiety item anxious ideas (presentiments), weak significance (≤0.05) for ability to relax and restlessness and for the depression items only feeling held back differed significantly; no other item was even weakly significant. The median for anxiety was not significantly different in the two subpopulations, while the median for depression was weakly significant (p=0.02).

Reliability and Validity of the FAQ

Internal consistency of the original, entire tiredness assessment questionnaire was examined with the Cronbach's alpha test and revealed a high reliability coefficient of 0.88. Reliability of the subscales as defined by factor analysis was confirmed for the factor 1 items with a reliability estimate of 0.84 (Tables 6, 7).

The items of the questionnaire had been derived from interviews with cancer patients and healthy individuals, and content validity was therefore supported by the fact that items reflected the true experience of those concerned. Content validity was also supported by the significant differences between cancer patients and healthy individuals on specific items, sensitively reflecting the "unusual tiredness" items and "healthy tiredness" items (Tables 2, 3). No other comparable validated instrument was available for use as an external criterion to examine convergent and concurrent validity. Criterion-related validity of the questionnaire was supported by the differences shown in results obtained in the two different health statuses in healthy and diseased individuals (Tables 2, 3, 8). Cross-correlation of items related to the time span of measurement revealed the higher phi coefficients for the measurement periods of today and last week (Table 4) and supported the appropriateness of the measurement periods today and last week.

Discussion

Qualitative Data as a Valid Foundation of the Study

This study, designed with the purpose of developing an instrument to measure tiredness/fatigue in cancer patients that would be applicable for epidemiological research, was an ambitious project. As knowledge gained from experience and from the literature was not sufficient to allow the planned research to be reliably conducted, previous research with qualitative research methods was first needed to explore valid descriptors of tiredness. The expert knowledge gained from a previous qualitative interview study with cancer patients and healthy individuals (Glaus 1996) was therefore used to build the foundation for this research project. As interviews are a form of self-report, the researcher can assume that the information given by an interviewee is accurate. However, the quality of data generated by this type of qualitative research has been described as largely dependent on the skills and expertise of the interviewer (Guba and Lincoln 1981). These aspects were considered with great care, and issues of rigor were addressed in the previously described qualitative study.

Composition of the Questionnaire Items from Responses of Cancer Patients and Healthy Individuals

The construction of the questionnaire first involved reduction of redundant items derived from the previous interview study, in which some items were equally observed in healthy individuals and in cancer patients; many, however, turned out to be specific to one group or the other. Items that were found in both groups were therefore unified for the questionnaire, but all group-specific items were retained with the aim of detecting cancer-specific fatigue. It could be argued that specific items in the group of healthy individuals could have been omitted from the questionnaire. This was not done, because the possible absence of items reflecting "healthy fatigue" would show what was not occurring in cancer patients; thus the absence of the expression of "healthy tiredness" would sharpen the picture of fatigue in cancer patients.

This strategy was supported by the results of this study. The delineation of cancer-specific tiredness was made more evident by the differences between the two groups. For example, the items decreased physical performance and weakness were significantly more strongly represented in cancer patients, whereas pleasant tiredness and heavy legs were significantly more strongly represented in healthy individuals (Table 2). Pleasant tiredness even showed minus values for cancer patients (Tables 2, 5). It turned out to be a privilege of healthy persons to feel pleasantly tired. This knowledge brings up the question as to whether activity, such as physical exercise, could change the type of tiredness experienced by diseased persons. This activity/rest balance pattern will be related to theory later in the discussion.

Comparison of Questionnaire Content with Items of Instruments Described in the Literature

There is a difference in the description of tiredness between existing measurement instruments and the items in the new questionnaire. Whereas scales derived by psychologists, such as the POMS scale (McNair and Lorr 1971), use descriptions derived from psychology, quality of life measures, such as the EORTC questionnaire (Hürny and Bernhard 1993), include descriptions related to wellness/illness and symptoms. A questionnaire developed by a nurse mainly assesses the impact and consequences of fatigue (Piper 1992). This reveals that the purpose of measuring fatigue is most important and that the instrument must fit the research purpose. The description of fatigue in tired airmen (Pearson and Byars 1956) differs considerably from what is experienced as fatigue in cancer patients. In contrast, a cancer-specific instrument would not be sufficiently sensitive to assess tiredness in healthy airmen. In this light, the decision to identify the descriptions of fatigue in cancer patients by means of interviews supports the content validity of the questionnaire for the purpose of the intended study. For example, no other instrument asks about decreased physical performance, which turned out to be a prominent feature of fatigue in the cancer population under study. The instrument had first of all to reflect the true experience of fatigue in cancer patients.

Age, Gender, and Disease Characteristics

It was reported some years ago that age and gender accounted for the variance of symptoms and that younger patients were more likely to report fatigue (Nerenz and Leventhal 1982). This factor was excluded, because age and gender were equally distributed in the study. The group of cancer patients consisted of a severely ill population with a wide variety of cancer types, mainly in advanced stages, and most of these patients were undergoing chemotherapy. Results obtained from a specific cancer population in only one stage of disease and with only one type of treatment might have shown different results. As the aim was to develop a questionnaire for use in a general cancer population, it seemed appropriate to include a general cancer patient population in the study.

Univariate and Multivariate Discrimination of Items Between Cancer Patients and Healthy Individuals in Three Time Spans

Concerning the time span today, mainly physical descriptions of tiredness and general indicators of tiredness were significantly stronger in cancer patients than in healthy individuals (Table 2). Affective and cognitive expressions did not differ between the two groups. This could be explained by the fact that the time period of today is too short to assess cognitive and affective symptoms or that people do not want to disclose affective attitudes.

However, anxiety and impaired concentration increased in importance for the longer time span of one week, although other, mainly cognitive and affective, items remained insignificant in both groups. Anxiety even increased in significance over the time period of one month. This suggests that anxiety might be more of a trait measure (reaction without time frame) rather than a state measure (reaction within a time frame), as differentiated by Van Dam and Linssen (1984). Whether the affective signs remain undetected by the insensitivity of the tool or by the wish of people not to disclose such feelings to others remains to be uncovered by further studies. Findings of other researchers have also suggested that patients may have less difficulty in expressing physical problems than emotional distress (Kobashi and Hanewald 1985). The correlation of tiredness with anxiety/depression levels, as measured with the HAD Scale (Tables 9, 10) in this study, also showed rather low correlations, and only one item of the depression scale differed significantly between cancer patients and healthy individuals (Table 10). A further explanation for this lack of difference between the two groups could be a true lack of difference between the groups in anxiety and depression, which from clinical experience is difficult to accept. Findings of this study are controversial when compared with those of studies that detected correlations between mood disturbances and fatigue levels. Blesch and Paice (1991) described correlations of scores of the POMS subscales with self-reported fatigue scores in patients with breast and lung cancer. The question of whether anxiety and depression are more easily detected by the POMS scales than by the HAD scales therefore arises.

Decreased physical performance, unusual tiredness, weakness, sleepiness in the daytime, unusual need for rest, fight to overcome inactivity, becoming slower, loss of energy, and general unwellness remained highly significant in cancer patients in all time spans. This can be explained by the fact that overall values in these items were very high in this study group. It supports the predominance of these physical items in the concept of fatigue in cancer patients.

Surprisingly, exhaustion did not appear to be more relevant in either of the two groups. Experience suggests it is possible that exhaustion is a feeling that appears following intensive physical activity in healthy persons and at the very end of advanced disease. No majority of either group filled out the assessment form after intensive physical exercise or at the very end of life. In this sense, exhaustion can be seen as the end of the fatigue continuum, with different meanings for diseased and healthy individuals. It suggests that for healthy persons exhaustion equals pleasant tiredness experienced after physical stress, and for cancer patients it equals highest intensity of tiredness experienced as distress and with a life-limiting impact.

According to the results of the logistic regression analysis (Table 3), some items appeared to be redundant. This could be explained by the fact that the inter-relationships between some items were very close, reflecting very similar concepts. Unusual, extreme tiredness might be equal to unusual need for rest or to unusual need for sleep or loss of energy or general unwellness. The concepts appear very similar, having a general impact on individuals. In order to conceptualize fatigue and to analyze its components, all items will be retained in the questionnaire for further analysis.

Reliability of the Time Frame of Measurement

The time span of today seemed inappropriate for the measurement of tiredness. Healthy persons experienced more pleasant tiredness in the time span of last week than they did for the time span of today. This can be explained by the high probability for healthy individuals to have had a hard working day or an intensive physical activity during last week, which is less probable for the time span of today, especially if the measurement is being taken in the morning. This supports the choice of a 1-week measurement period for critical items. Some other critical items in this tool, especially for cancer patients, were feeling sleepy during the daytime, unusual need for rest, and exhaustion, again especially if measurement was being taken in the morning.

The highest correlation was seen between the results obtained for the time spans today and last week. This period paid regard to the fluctuating construct of tiredness, which might differ from one day to the next. The 1-week period seemed less affected by unusual short-term events. However, treatment variables need to be controlled to obtain valid results for a specific measurement purpose. In cancer patients, treatment and treatment-rest periods might induce relevant differences, as observed by other researchers, who concluded that peak levels of fatigue could well have been found at another time period than at the actual time of measurement (Pickard-Holley 1991). This underlines the importance of controlling confounding variables such as treatment strategies.

The theoretical justification of the time frame by the differentiation between state and trait measures (Huismann and van Dam 1987) has been described above. From this study it can be suggested that tiredness itself represents a mixture of trait and state measure. It might be more of a state measure after chemo- or radiotherapy but might be rather a trait measure if tiredness is related to tumor activity over longer periods of time.

The lower phi coefficient values were found between the time span of today and last month, indicating that the remembered severity of the symptoms might decline with increasing duration of the time span the lesser be remembered. Memory effects on validity of data might be crucial (Van Dam and Linssen 1984).

Intensity of Tiredness, Resultant Distress, and Their Correlation with Other Variables

The continuum of tiredness in other studies was defined with "I do not feel tired" to "I feel completely exhausted" (Holmes 1991; McCorkle and Young 1978; Piper and Lindsey 1989). The LASA scales in this study, describing the continuum "I did not experience unusual tiredness" to "I felt completely exhausted," and also the distress resulting from tiredness, were found to be sensitive and reliable, as the difference between healthy individuals and cancer patients was significant (Table 8). Use of the term "unusual tiredness," to ensure the ascertainment of tiredness that exceeds normal diurnal tiredness, was considered an appropriate way to address fatigue in cancer patients, as it was identified in the study described in the chapter "A Qualitative Study to Explore the Concept of Fatigue/Tiredness in Cancer Patients and in Healthy Individuals."

Correlation between the Karnofsky Index and tiredness intensity and between the Karnovsky Index and the level of distress caused by tiredness was very low, which may be explained by the fact that 86% of the patient population had Karnofsky Index scores higher than 80. Again, no correlation was found between the results of the HAD Scale and tiredness, except for the difference between study groups on the Depression item "feeling held back" (Table 1).

Reliability and Validity of the Questionnaire

Reliability was confirmed for the entire tiredness questionnaire. Satisfactory reliability was confirmed for the subscale with physical tiredness items. Even though reliability coefficients were lower for the cognitive and affective factors, the study suggests the need for further research to identify the source and impact of affective and cognitive signs. Identification or rejection of further subscales needs to be supported in a study with a larger population. Validity concerning content has been established by significant discrimination of instrument items between cancer patients and healthy individuals and by the use of items derived from self-reports from the populations concerned. Investigation of the time frames has confirmed the reliable use of the time span of the past week.

Contribution to the Understanding of Fatigue in Cancer Patients

Using Factor Analysis as a Hypothesis-Generating Technique

Factor analyses were carried out to examine construct validity and to identify sub scales and possible unified concepts. Factor 1 (Table 7) was confirmed with satisfactory reliability. Again, this cluster comprised mainly physical items, apart from loss of interest. Loss of interest seems a logical consequence of decreased physical capacity and reduced activity. Here it becomes clear that psychological reactions are interwoven with physical experiences. The items of factor 2, representing only affective and cognitive aspects, had higher reliability than factor 3, which unified pleasant tiredness with exhaustion and heavy limbs, yielding another kind of physical tiredness sensations, which should possibly be seen as a decrease in physical capacity. Results of factor analysis suggested that there was a clear physical component inherent and predominant in tiredness, and that affective and cognitive items were involved, but that there was no clear knowledge to support the hypothesis of a physical, affective and cognitive model of expression of tiredness. Even though this categorization was similarly described by others (Yoshitake 1971), it must be treated with caution, because confounding variables might be involved. It could be argued that an affective expression of tiredness, such as sadness, might be an expression of the whole situation, and that sadness is more a sign of depression resulting from the life-threatening circumstances than an expression of tiredness. The concept of physical, affective and cognitive tiredness needs to be further examined.

Researchers who developed similar subscales guided by factor analysis were Kobashi and Hanewald (1985) and Chalder and Berelowitz (1993). Kobashi identified a physical fatigue scale, a mental fatigue scale and a general condition scale when he examined patients undergoing radiotherapy. The physical scale does not include weakness or decreased physical performance, but rather includes the items derived from the Yoshitake symptom checklist

(Yoshitake 1971), which was developed for a healthy working population (Kobashi and Hanewald 1985). Chalder developed a physical and a mental scale, examining patients in a general practice setting. The physical scale concurs with some of the physical signs in this study, including rest, sleepiness, weakness. However, the validity of questionnaire items can be questioned if they are derived from populations other than cancer patients and if they are generated solely by professionals.

In this study, factor analysis points to unified concepts within the instrument, and these can help to develop the understanding of the construct under test. The physical expressions of tiredness were prominent, and the question is whether the measurement of the physical items, included here in factor 1, would be sufficient in a fatigue measurement instrument for cancer patients. However, the affective and cognitive aspects, unified in factor 2, cannot be disregarded, and together with the content validity given by cancer-patient-generated items, this study suggests that the nonphysical items should be included in the questionnaire. In further research with a larger cancer-patient population, factor analysis will give more information on the quality of fatigue in cancer patients. In order to achieve this, evaluations will need to target qualitative aspects in addition to intensity or quantity of tiredness. This seems especially important for directing the future development of supportive strategies.

An Evolving Hypothesis: The Vicious Circle Phenomenon of Activity/Inactivity. A Major Physical Concept of Tiredness in Cancer Patients?

The clear identification of physical expressions of tiredness leads to the need for further theory development. In this study, the unusual need for rest turned out to be a strong, cancer-specific expression of tiredness measured in all time spans (Table 2). The need to rest seemed to contradict the hypothesis that exercise relieves tiredness (Winningham and Nail 1994). Results of this study suggest that there could be a vicious circle (Fig. 1): unusual tiredness leading to an unusual need for rest, which, in turn, leads to weakness, which then leads to decreased physical performance, to problems in overcoming inactivity, to unusual tiredness and so forth. Becoming slower, loss of energy, loss of interest and general unwellness could be seen as inherent and also as vicious-circle-type consequences of this activity/rest imbalance. The question as to whether it might be possible to interrupt this circle by exercise or whether this predetermined circle cannot be interrupted as long as the original cause of tiredness, such as cancer or treatment measures, cannot be eliminated remains open.

It was found that in a research-based nursing rehabilitation program, the nonexercise group reported twice the fatigue intensity reported by the exercise group (Mock and Burke, in press). However, are such programs applicable to patients with adjuvant chemotherapy as well as to those with advanced disease, and to what cancer populations can they safely be offered? Which

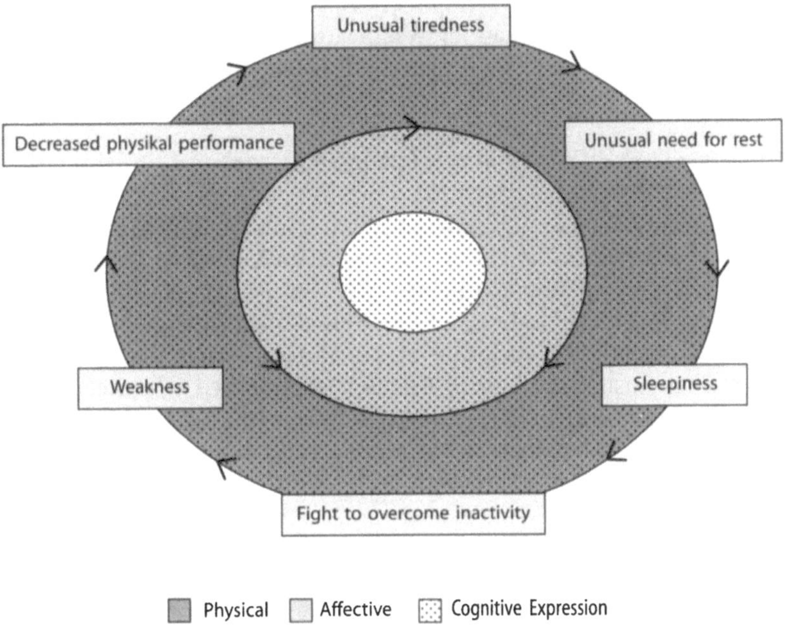

Fig. 1. The activity/rest imbalance in fatigue: a vicious circle?

measurement instrument will allow reliable measurement of success or failure? The frequently used POMS (McNair and Lorr 1971) measures psychological expression of tiredness, but it remains to be substantiated whether physical exercise induces relief from depression or relief from physical tiredness. This cannot be assessed by scales that do not explicitly measure physical as well as psychological tiredness symptoms.

The Winningham's Psychobiological-Entropy Model, a theoretical concept of fatigue (Fig. 5 in the chapter entitled "The Concept of Fatigue or Tiredness as Experienced In Health and Disease, and More Specifically in Cancer"), emphasizes the need to determine the optimal balance between restorative rest and restorative activity or exercise. Part of the model relates fatigue to activity and functioning (Winningham and Nail 1994). However, caution about the use of exercise has been reported, owing to the extremely complex and mainly unknown mechanisms of fatigue in cancer patients (Winningham 1991; St. Pierre and Kaspar 1992). The hypothesis of a vicious circle of activity/inactivity derived from this study fits the theoretical energy deficit concept of Winningham. However, it can only be one concept influencing the production of tiredness, as many further potential causes and etiologic factors, as described in the theoretical model by Piper (1993), might play a part. The results from this study give these influencing factors a new weighting, in the sense that tiredness is strongly associated with activity and rest patterns, which are primarily determined by physical sources. Whether the affective and cognitive responses can be seen as specific expressions of tiredness in cancer patients or whether they should be seen as general expressions of the overall disease situation is not yet clear.

Conclusions and Directions for Further Research

A tiredness assessment questionnaire has been developed to analyze the experience of tiredness/fatigue in cancer patients. The items for the questionnaire were derived from interviews with cancer patients and healthy individuals and considered to be valid descriptors of how fatigue is experienced by those concerned. The inclusion of descriptors derived from healthy individuals distinguished the type of tiredness experienced in cancer patients, thus reflecting the absence of health-specific expressions of tiredness. Some new items, which are not included as signs or expressions of tiredness in available questionnaires or scales, were identified in the interviews and integrated in the new FAQ.

The use of the new instrument FAQ in this study with 77 healthy individuals and 77 cancer patients allowed reliability and validity tests and contributed to a theory of fatigue. A previous framework, which classified the expressions of fatigue as physical, affective and cognitive expressions, was completed with the finding that the physical expression of fatigue might be more dominant than affective and cognitive expressions. The physical dominance of fatigue in cancer patients was presented as decreased physical performance, unusual tiredness, weakness, sleepiness in the daytime, unusual need for rest, fight to overcome inactivity, becoming slower, loss of energy and general unwellness. These signs of fatigue were tentatively summarized and put forward as a physical component of fatigue. A hypothesis was formulated, presenting this component as a vicious circle phenomenon involving an imbalance between rest and activity. Although it suggests that tiredness in cancer patients is expressed at physical, affective and cognitive levels, the results of the study argue for a high weighting of the physical expression.

Investigation of the time frame of measurement of tiredness indicated that the use of the time span last week may be the most valid and reliable time frame. Intensity of and distress caused by tiredness, as measured with a linear analogue scale, showed significant differences between the two study populations, which supports the validity of the definition of the tiredness continuum distinguishing tiredness from unusual tiredness.

Reliability and validity of the questionnaire as a measurement instrument for the experience of tiredness in cancer patients, including its feasibility and acceptability by this vulnerable population, have been supported. For the purpose of an epidemiological research project in cancer patients, the instrument needs small adaptations, such as the inclusion of a few further items for affective and cognitive signs, as derived from the interviews, in order to facilitate further investigation of the theoretical framework using the factor analysis technique. Randomization of the items to determine the sequence of items in the questionnaire is needed, to prevent researcher-induced sequence-bias. Use of the measurement period "one week" can be practiced confidently. The limited number of 22 questionnaire items with dichotomous answers, related to the measurement for one time span, will allow its use in further studies with large populations with limited energy. After a first, successful, development period, the FAQ will be used for further research with the aim of identifying groups of cancer patients at risk, and eventually for evaluation of therapeutic strategies. At the same time, further studies mean continuation of the validation process of the questionnaire.

References

Blesch K, Paice J (1991) Correlates of fatigue in breast or lung cancer. Oncol Nurs Forum 18:81–87

Bortz J (1985) Lehrbuch der Statistik für Sozialwissenschaftler. Springer, Berlin Heidelberg New York

Chalder T, Berelowitz T (1993) Development of a fatigue scale. J Psychosom Res 37 (2):147–153

Field P, Morse J (1985) Nursing research. The application of qualitative approaches. Chapman and Hall, London

Glaus A (1996) A qualitative study to explore the concept of fatigue/tiredness in cancer patients and in healthy individuals. Support Care Cancer 4:82–96

Guba E, Lincoln J (1981) Effective evaluation. Jossey-Bass, San Francisco

Herrmann C, Scholz K (1991) Psychologisches Screening von Patienten einer kardiologischen Akutklinik mit einer deutschen Fassung der Hospital Anxiety and Depression (HAD) Skala. Psychother Psychosom Med Psychol 41:83–92

Holmes S (1991) Preliminary investigation of symptom distress in two cancer patient populations: evaluation of a measurement instrument. J Adv Nurs 16:439–446

Huisman S, van Dam F (1987) On measuring complaints of cancer patients: some remarks on the time span question. In: Aaronson N, Beckmann J (eds) The quality of life of cancer patients. Raven, New York

Hürny C, Bernhard J (1993) Fatigue and malaise as quality of life indicator in small-cell lung cancer patients. Support Care Cancer 1:316–320

Jones D, Feyers P, Simons J, et al (1987) Measuring and analysing quality of life in cancer clinical trials: a review. In: Aaronson N, Beckmann J (eds) The quality of life in cancer patients. Raven, New York, pp 41–61

Karnofsky D, Burchenal J (1949) Clinical evaluation of chemotherapeutic agents in cancer. In: Macleod C (ed) Evaluation of chemotherapeutic agents. Columbia University Press, New York

Kobashi J, Hanewald G (1985) Assessment of malaise in cancer patients treated with radiotherapy. Cancer Nurs 12:306–313

McCorkle R, Young K (1978) Development of a symptom distress scale. Cancer Nurs 10:373–378

McNair D, Lorr M (1971) EITS manual for the profile f mood states. Educational and Industrial Testing Service, San Diego

Mock V, Burke M (in press) A nursing rehabilitation programme for women with breast cancer on adjuvant chemotherapy. Oncol Nurs Forum

Nerenz D, Leventhal H (1982) Factors contributing to emotional distress during cancer chemotherapy. Cancer 50:1020–1027

Nigel G (1993) Analyzing tabular data. UCL, London

Oppenheim A (1992) Questionnaire design, interviewing and attitude measurement. Pinter, London

Pearson P, Byars G (1956) The development and validation of a checklist measuring subjective fatigue (report no 56–115). School of Aviation, Randolph AFB, TX
Pickard-Holley S (1991) Fatigue in cancer patients. Cancer Nurs 14 (1):13–19
Piper B (1992) Subjective fatigue in women receiving six cycles of adjuvant chemotherapy for breast cancer. PhD dissertation, University of California, San Francisco. Ann Arbor, MI: UMI Dissertation Services (no 9303553)
Piper B (1993) Fatigue. In: Carrieri V, Lindsey A (eds) Pathophysiological phenomena in nursing: human response to illness. Saunders, Philadelphia
Piper B, Lindsey A (1989) The development of an instrument to measure the subjective dimension of fatigue. In: Funk S, Tornquist A (eds) Key aspects of comfort. Springer, Berlin Heidelberg New York
Polit D, Hungler B (1993) Nursing research, principles and methods. Lippincott, Philadelphia
Schag C, Heinrich R (1984) Karnofsky performance status revisited: reliability, validity and guidelines. J Clin Oncol 2 (3):187–193
St Pierre P, Kaspar C (1992) Fatigue mechanisms in patients with cancer: effects of tumour necrosis factor and exercise on skeletal muscle. Oncol Nurs Forum 19:419–425
Van Dam F, Linssen A (1984) Evaluating quality of life: behavioural measures in clinical trials. In: Buyse M, Staquet M (eds) Cancer clinical trials: method and practice. Oxford University Press, New York
Winningham M (1991) Walking programme for people with cancer: Getting started. Cancer Nurs 14:270–276
Winningham M, Nail M (1994) Fatigue and the cancer experience: the state of the knowledge. Oncol Nurs Forum 21 (1):23–36
Yoshitake H (1971) Relations between the symptoms and feelings of fatigue. Ergonomics 14:175–186
Zigmond A, Snaith R (1983) The Hospital Anxiety and Depression Scale. Acta Psychiatr Scand 67:361–370

The Relationship Between Fatigue and Type and Stage of Cancer

Introduction

The previous chapters of this book have shown that the concept of tiredness/fatigue is still ill defined. Its qualitative exploration in the chapter "A Qualitative Exploration of the Concept of Fatigue/Tiredness in Cancer Patients and in Healthy Individuals" gave new insight into the experience of fatigue. The comparison of these findings with concepts in existing measurement instruments showed a lack of valid instruments for epidemiological fatigue research in cancer patients and eventually led to the construction of the new Fatigue Assessment Questionnaire (FAQ), which was then tested in cancer patients and healthy individuals. The next study now attempts to measure the relationship of fatigue in cancer patients with different types and stages of cancer, using this new FAQ. At the same time, the study allows a further validation process of FAQ in a larger cancer patient population.

Review of the Literature

Fatigue and tiredness have become frequent research topics in recent years. Tiredness and exhaustion seem to be attributes of modern society. The biological meaning and aim of tiredness, as described by the fatigue theorist Grandjean (1968), lies in the fact that nature guides the behavior of humans and animals through feelings of fatigue to help the body to find its balance between rest and activity, thus being a life-sustaining state similar to other physiological needs, such as thirst or hunger. It is difficult, however, to capture tiredness that is in the process of evolving from a "healthy, life-sustaining state" into a life-distressing sign or symptom of an approaching disaster or breakdown. This has become especially clear during recent years, when the new diagnosis "chronic fatigue syndrome" (CFS) has stirred up a great deal of controversy (Greenberg 1990). Is it a disease, a postviral syndrome or a sign of psychological disorders? Apart from tiredness in the CFS, tiredness itself cannot be seen as a disease and occurs in healthy as well as in diseased individuals.

Differences Between Baseline Data of Healthy Individuals and Cancer Patients

To determine the significance of tiredness as a sign of physical or psychological distress, the identification of baseline levels and experience of tiredness in healthy individuals is required. Data collected during a large survey (1971–1974) of more than 2000 American adults between 25 and 74 years of age were used to explore self-perceived fatigue. Fourteen percent of these men and 20% of the women reported suffering from fatigue (Chen 1986). This means that the prevalence of fatigue in cancer patients should be higher than that, in order to justify the conclusion that cancer patients differ in their fatigue experience from the general population. It is unknown whether results from that time period can be compared with the fatigue experience of today.

So far, most cancer fatigue research projects have failed to include a control group. A study by Irvine et al. (1994) compared the fatigue experience of 104 cancer patients, mainly women with breast cancer, who were undergoing chemotherapy and radiotherapy with the fatigue experience of 53 healthy women. The first measurement was taken before the beginning of therapy, and at this time point no significant difference was found between breast cancer patients and healthy individuals. Levels of fatigue, however, increased in the course of treatment in cancer patients and were then significantly higher than in the healthy population. The lack of difference between the two study populations before the start of treatment poses the question as to whether breast cancer itself is a non-fatigue-inducing type of cancer. In a further study, investigating fatigue in 12 patients with ovarian cancer, no significant difference was found in comparison with 12 healthy women (Pickard-Holley 1991). This lack of difference may be explained by the small sample or may be related to ovarian cancer as a non-fatigue-inducing cancer.

Even though it has been difficult so far to demonstrate that healthy individuals experience less fatigue than cancer patients without treatment, it can be hypothesized that the quality of tiredness might be more distressing in disease than in health. A study comparing fatigue levels over daily periods in 30 healthy persons and 20 cancer patients suggested different tiredness profiles with different impacts (Glaus 1993). Whereas cancer patients experienced distressing tiredness all day long, healthy persons experienced pleasant tiredness in the evening only. Again, a mixed cancer population and small sample size limit the generalizability of these results.

In the study conducted to test the validity and reliability of the FAQ, 77 cancer patients, most with advanced cancer, who were receiving chemotherapy and 77 healthy individuals documented their tiredness and the distress it was causing them on linear analogue scales. The median intensity of and distress caused by tiredness was significantly higher in the group of cancer patients for the time periods of today, last week and last month than in the group of healthy individuals (see Table 8 in the chapter on "Testing the Fatigue Assessment Questionnaire in Healthy Persons and in Cancer Patients"). These findings support the notion that there is a difference between cancer patients and healthy individuals in baseline fatigue values, but the heterogeneity of patients with a wide variety of tumor types and treatments made it difficult to identify baseline fatigue data for cancer patients with specific types of cancer.

Fatigue and Its Relationship to Type and Stage of Cancer

Clinical experience suggests that there is a relationship between different types of cancer and fatigue. Hürny and Bernhard (1993) demonstrated that 43% of 83 small cell lung cancer patients suffered from fatigue before the initiation of chemotherapy. Intensity of tiredness decreased only very little during six cycles of chemotherapy, in contrast to cough, which decreased significantly during treatment, thus indicating successful treatment (Hürny and Bernhard 1993). It might be suggested that if lung cancer itself were the cause of fatigue, fatigue would also have decreased with successful cancer treatment. It could also be possible, however, that chemotherapy had caused the fatigue. An investigation in 69 women with non-small-cell lung cancer (limited disease) prior to treatment indicated that 59% of them suffered from reduced energy (Sarna 1994). Reduced energy was demonstrated in difficulties with household chores (33%) and interference with work (28%). Three quarters of the patients were not satisfied with their level of activities. The fact that women in this study had limited disease and that they were untreated when the assessment took place suggests very strongly that the type of cancer (lung cancer) is responsible for the development of fatigue distress. Blesch and Paice (1991) found no significant difference between chemotherapy-treated patients with lung and breast cancer: two thirds of the patients in both groups experienced moderate to severe fatigue. It is not possible to identify whether fatigue in these patients was induced by the disease or by the treatment. In another study, high levels of tiredness were observed in patients with head and neck cancer (very small subsample) and in breast cancer, using the GLQ-8, an eight-item LASA instrument, to measure specific side effects of cancer and cancer treatment (Butow and Coates 1991). However, the lack of balanced disease groups, the variety of treatment interventions and the small numbers in the subgroups diminish the relevance of the study.

Fatigue and Type of Cancer: Are There Specific Tumors that Produce Asthenins?

It has been proposed that the malignant process itself may secrete substances that cause asthenia (Theologides 1982). Asthenia has been defined as pathologic fatiguability, loss of strength and generalized weakness (Bruera 1988), which can be seen as major components of fatigue. A further hypothesis that is discussed is the promotion of a defense mechanism of the body against the tumor, in the course of which cytokines, such as interferons, interleukins and tumor necrosis factors (TNF), may be secreted and so induce fatigue

(Morant 1991). A study with 87 non-small-cell lung cancer patients tested whether metabolic derangements were related to a systematic inflammatory response. Increase in energy expenditure, weight loss and plasma levels of different TNF were measured. Tumor stage was found to be significantly different between weight-losing and weight-stable patients, and levels of inflammatory mediators were increased (Staal-van den Brekel and Dentener 1995). It could be argued that weight loss induced by tumor growth involves fatigue and therefore inflammatory mediators are co-responsible for its development. As inflammatory mediators seem to be tumor specific, the correlation of fatigue with specific types of cancer can be suggested from this viewpoint.

Increased rates of energy expenditure and cachexia in cancer patients might be related to such immunological processes (Keller 1993) and may further increase fatigue. From a study aimed at testing the effect of specific tumor types on neuromuscular function in rats, it was concluded that the development of neuromyopathy was more intensive in rats with Guérin epithelioma than in rats with fibrosarcoma. These results supported the hypothesis of a hormonal influence of the neoplasm on the neuromuscular system. These results were compared with clinical observations in tumor patients; an overall reduction of sensory excitability was noted in different patients, and a decrease of the general myoelectrical activity was observed (Koczocik and Krzysztof 1994). This kind of research may advance our knowledge about fatigue and the detection of new substances, which could at least partially account for the development of fatigue in specific types of tumors.

Several of the publications discussed suggest inflammatory mediators and/or immunological processes as potential causes of fatigue in cancer patients. In contrast, a recent study suggested that the CFS was associated with an increased susceptibility to cancer. Data from a cancer registry in the United States of America were reviewed subsequent to a reported outbreak of a CFS-like illness between 1984 and 1986, concentrating on non-Hodgkin lymphoma and brain tumors. An upward trend in the incidence of brain tumors, which could be related to a national upward trend for this disease, was noted (Levine and Atherton 1994). This was not the case for patients with non-Hodgkin lymphoma. Methodological difficulties were considered. Further studies are needed to investigate possible associations between CFS and cancer, including expected latent periods for specific tumors. This interesting theory looks at fatigue as a cause or precursor of cancer, while most current studies have looked at fatigue as a consequence of disease and treatment. The relationship between specific tumor types and fatigue could be suggested as a linking factor between the two theories.

New substances have been detected in recent years, which are now being tested in patients with fatigue. A pilot test of physiological fatigue indicators in 15 healthy controls showed the correlation of rising salivary melatonin levels in the evening and nighttime hours with a corresponding decline in body temperature (Anderson and Dean 1996). It suggests that melatonin, a neurotransmitter associated with the sleep/wake cycle, also has an influence on fatigue in cancer patients. Whether different types and stages of disease play a part in the production of melatonin needs to be further examined. From the interventional viewpoint, promising hypotheses could be tested.

The Influence of Other Symptoms on Fatigue in Patients with Cancer

Today, fatigue is recognized as the most common and probably most distressing symptom reported by cancer patients, even though methodological problems and differences in measurement make it difficult to compare available research (Holmes 1991; World Health Organisation 1990; Piper and Lindsey 1989; McCorkle and Young 1978). A recent study investigating the incidence and severity of symptoms in 1000 patients with advanced cancer showed that fatigue, together with pain and anorexia, was consistently among the 10 most prevalent symptoms (Donelli and Walsh 1995). This study supports the idea that tiredness correlates with advanced stages of cancer, but it does not differentiate between types of tumors. It has been hypothesized that there is an interrelationship between symptoms and that fatigue, as a primary symptom of disease or treatment, leads to secondary fatigue by way of decreased activity as a consequence of other symptoms, such as pain and immobility (Winningham et al. 1994). This could explain the high incidence of fatigue, especially in advanced disease and when intensive treatment with side effects is involved.

Another study showed that the numbers of symptoms and fatigue in cancer patients before chemotherapy were significant predictors when outcomes were analyzed individually in 229 cancer patients (Jones 1994). This study emphasizes that fatigue is a pretreatment symptom, which supports the hypothesis that fatigue is associated with type and stage of cancer. However, in this study fatigue was measured with subscales of the POMS (McNair and Lorr 1971), which might represent measurement of mood states, possibly associated with uncertainty and anxiety before the start of cancer treatment, rather than measurement of multidimensional fatigue.

The Influence of Treatment Effects on Fatigue

Interesting observations have been made on the development of fatigue in patients with different tumors during therapy. Fatigue levels in patients with lung cancer were observed to be higher before and during radiotherapy than after (Haylock and Hart 1979). One explanation tentatively proposed is that the decrease in tumor burden results in lower fatigue levels owing to better oxygen exchange, less respiratory distress or reduced production of cytokines. In contrast, patients with localized breast cancer who were receiving adjuvant radiotherapy experienced higher levels of fatigue after treatment than before (Kobashi et al. 1985). This may be explained by the fact that there was no primary tumor bulk to be reduced by the treatment, but that patients experienced fatigue as side effects of adjuvant radiotherapy. It could be concluded that palliative radiotherapy can reduce fatigue, especially if the functional capacity of the organ concerned can be increased by the treatment, and that adjuvant radiotherapy might increase fatigue, because these patients have no tumor burden and have a good general condition, but experience side effects of the treatment. This would support the idea that fatigue can be correlated with type and stage of the disease, but that in different situations different causes of fatigue need to be distinguished.

The Influence of Treatment Side Effects on Fatigue

Fatigue is known as one of the few systemic side effects of radiation therapy. It has been found to increase towards the end of treatment (King and Nail 1985; Haylock and Hart 1979). In many studies investigating fatigue in relation to chemotherapy, fatigue has been demonstrated to be the most prevalent side effect (Blesch and Paice 1991; Rhodes and Watson 1988; Knoff 1986; Meyerowitz and Watkins 1983; Nerenz and Leventhal 1982). An increase has been observed with progression of therapy (Love and Leventhal 1989). Investigations of fatigue in patients with different chemotherapy regimens indicated similar fatigue levels among groups receiving different chemotherapy regimens (Richardson 1996). A very recent study in 715 women with localized breast cancer showed that fatigue scores were highest among those receiving a combination of radiotherapy and chemotherapy (Woo and Dipple 1996). Fatigue has been seen as the dose-limiting factor of treatment with biotherapy (Piper and Rieger 1989). These and many further studies show that the influence of cancer treatment is an important factor in fatigue. As it would be unrealistic and undesirable to reduce or even omit cancer treatment because of fatigue, it will be important to provide cancer patients undergoing different treatment regimens with anticipatory guidance. However, a challenge in future studies will be the identification of the underlying causes of fatigue, as there are no baseline data that indicate whether the type and stage of the disease, or the treatment, or both, are ultimately responsible for fatigue. This knowledge is needed to develop scientifically based interventional strategies.

The Possible Influence of Coping with Cancer on Fatigue

Clinical experience shows that coping with a life-threatening disease involves feelings of sadness and anxiety. Positive correlations between fatigue, sadness and anxiety in cancer patients have been established (Blesch and Paice 1991; Bruera and Brenneis 1989). The question of whether fatigue is a symptom of the disease or an expression of coping, or both, cannot yet be answered. Looking at cancer as a life crisis, especially if the disease progresses, requires attention to the physical and biological changes as well as to the emotional aspects. It seems difficult to disentangle physical and emotional tiredness when disease is physically and emotionally overwhelming. Because of the interventional potential, it still remains important to analyze how far fatigue is rooted in emotional distress. Patients with different types of cancer in advanced stages might be at risk of experiencing fatigue not only physically but also emotionally, because of the effort needed to cope with the circumstances.

The Influence of the Measurement Instrument Selected on the Results of Fatigue Research in Cancer Patients

The lack of validated instruments to measure fatigue/tiredness in cancer patients has made it difficult to compare the results from available research. The frequently used vigor/fatigue scale of the POMS (McNair and Lorr 1971) measures fatigue mainly from a psychological viewpoint. Other instruments are too long and burdensome, not available in German (Piper and Lindsey 1989) or not constructed or validated for a cancer population (Yoshitake 1971; Pearson and Byars 1956). The new FAQ, developed from the cancer patients' perspective, measuring fatigue from the physical, affective and cognitive dimension (in the German language), was therefore now to be used for the first time in the epidemiological study described below, which at the same time would permit further validation of this new instrument. The instrument is described under the "Methods" section of this chapter, and its adapted, final version is presented in the Appendix (in the original German and translated into English; please note that the English translation has not yet been professionally translated and validated).

Aim of the Study

The aim of this study was to test the hypothesis that levels and expressions of fatigue correlate more with certain types of cancer than with others and that fatigue is more prominent and distressing in advanced and active cancer disease than in limited and inactive cancer. This multivariate hypothesis predicts a relationship between the type and stage of cancer and fatigue, which is deduced from the theory that fatigue is a multidimensional concept with a dominant biochemical, disease-related cause, as proposed earlier (see chapter on "Testing the Fatigue Assessment Questionnaire in Healthy Persons and in Cancer Patients").

At the same time, this hypothesis-testing study represented a further validation process for the new FAQ and was also intended to test the reliability and validity in a larger cancer patient population.

Research Approach, Setting, Patient Selection, and Study Population

The hypothesis was tested using a quantitative, explorative research approach. It had to be explorative because the baseline values in different cancer-patient populations were not known. Application of the FAQ in a large study population required a quantitative approach. It was an epidemiological cohort study, using a prospective, nonrandomized, cross-sectional study design. It had to be prospective because fatigue, a fluctuating, subjective state, could not be measured retrospectively. Randomization was not used because the study was explorative, although measures were taken to exclude selection bias. The cross-sectional design was chosen because of the aim of measuring the occurrence of fatigue epidemiologically in patients with specific tumor types. A descriptive and correlational approach was used to investigate the interrelationships among variables of interest.

The study was mainly conducted within the in- and outpatient services of the Medizinische Klinik C, Kantonsspital St. Gallen, Switzerland. During the last months of data collection, further patients were included from the departments of radio-oncology and gynecology of the same hospital, from a private oncology practice and from the oncology outpatient departments of two other hospitals. In total, four institutions were involved in the study. Patient accrual took place from October 1995 to June 1996.

Every patient admitted to the wards of the department was approached systematically within the first three days after admission to prevent diagnostic and therapeutic influences on the experience of fatigue. Every patient who visited the medical oncology outpatient department during a randomly selected time period (one day per week, rotating) was also asked to participate. This method was chosen to exclude selection bias, as the investigator was not available full-time for the study. Patients in the other adjacent institutions were selected according to the investigator's availability.

The study population included patients with the following types of cancer: breast cancer, lung cancer, malignant lymphoma (including myeloma), gastrointestinal cancer (including cancer of the esophagus, stomach, pancreas, gallbladder and liver), cancer of the ovaries and testicles, gynecological cancers (cervix, endometrium, vagina), melanoma and "other." This wide range of cancer disease types was selected so that the testing of the hypothesis could remain explorative. For this reason, power analyses to determine sample size were difficult, because there was uncertainty concerning baseline data.

Exclusion criteria were: (1) a diagnosis of brain tumor or known brain metastasis, because of their potential influence on the experience and perception of fatigue, (2) leukemia, because of the potential influence of acute blood disorders, infections and complications, and (3) cognitive impairment, psychiatric disorders and inability to understand and speak the German language.

Patients were not approached about entering the study if they had not been informed of a new diagnosis of cancer.

The study was approved by the ethical committee of the Kantonsspital St. Gallen. The medical and nursing directors of all departments and institutions involved confirmed their agreement with and support for the investigation.

Patients were asked by their caregivers to take part and had to give oral consent to involvement in the study. They were guaranteed confidentiality. Their names were kept on a separate list (to prevent a second approach), and the questionnaires were coded to ensure confidentiality.

Methods

Instruments

The FAQ

The new FAQ, developed at the Interdisciplinary Oncology Center in St. Gallen (see above), was used to assess expression and intensity of fatigue and the distress caused by it. This multidimensional, 22-item questionnaire (in German) concerning physical, affective and cognitive expression of fatigue is a self-assessment tool with dichotomous answers for measurement of fatigue in the time span of the previous week. Additional LASA scales for fatigue intensity and distress are included. This instrument was used because there was no other cancer-specific fatigue measurement instrument available that was short and easy to use, had been validated in the German language and was appropriate for epidemiological fatigue research in a large, diseased population vulnerable to fatigue. The items of the instrument were generated in previous, qualitative interviews with cancer patients and healthy individuals (see above), which supports content validity. Internal consistency was confirmed in an earlier study in cancer patients and in healthy individuals, and by then the scale showed an overall reliability coefficient of 0.88 (Cronbach's alpha), with a major physical subscale and a psychocognitive subscale (previous chapter). Before beginning with data analyses in this hypothesis-testing study, the FAQ was first factor-analyzed, again on the basis of the new and larger study population, and these results did provide theoretical underpinning for the construction of a physical, affective and cognitive subscale and suggested minor adaptations of the questionnaire. These adaptation processes are described later under "Psychometric Properties of the FAQ" in the "Results" section of this chapter. The final, adapted version of FAQ is presented in the Appendix (in German and translated into English).

The Hospital Anxiety and Depression Scale

This scale was originally developed to detect anxiety and depression in medical patients. Concepts of emotional and physical illness are separated, and evidence was presented that the scale scores were not affected by the presence of physical illness (Zigmond and Snaith 1983). The scale has been translated into the German language, and reliability and validity have been successfully established in patients with cardiac disease (Herrmann and Scholz 1991). The scale includes seven items concerning depression and seven items concerning anxiety, and relates to the time span of the previous week. This instrument was chosen because of its ability to distinguish between emotional and physical symptoms, which is especially important in a population with cancer. As it is not yet known whether fatigue is a physical symptom of the disease and its context or whether it is an expression of depression, it was the aim to detect anxiety and depression as separate concepts in relation to fatigue and to estimate their correlational occurrence.

The Karnofsky Index

The Karnofsky Index is a validated, numerical scale from 0 to 100 and represents the patient's ability to perform normal activity, the ability to do active work and the need for assistance in activities of daily living (Karnofsky and Abelmann 1949). Established guidelines for its use were considered; it has been widely tested and used as a basis for clinical decisions (Schag et al. 1984). This Index was considered to show correlations between activity status, stage of disease and tiredness, and the score was estimated by the researcher.

Patient Characteristics: Sociodemographic, Health-Related and Medical Data

Patients were asked to fill in a self-assessment form with questions about gender, age, self-perceived health status, cancer history, regular intake of medications, social context, employment situation and place of investigation. Additional medical data were collected by the investigator from the medical documents: date of diagnosis, type and stage of tumor at the time of investigation, tumor activity, tumor treatment within the last 6 weeks, other regular medications and in- or outpatient status. These data were needed to test the relationship between fatigue and disease so that the hypothesis could be tested.

Procedure

The research assistant and the nurses and doctors involved in this study first needed careful instruction to avoid introduction of any bias. As the questionnaire had already been tested before in the same institution, it could be used without further piloting. Patients were approached by their caregivers, who invited them to participate in the study. If they agreed to cooperate, they were approached individually by the researcher, who explained the study and asked for oral consent. Confidentiality was guaranteed, and the patients were instructed to fill out the forms in the following order: (a) the Fatigue Assessment Questionnaire (FAQ), (b) the HAD scale, and (c) the sociodemographic and health-related data. This sequence was chosen because it was thought that the form eliciting the sociodemographic data might discourage people from cooperating in the study. Most patients were left alone in a quiet place to fill out the questionnaires, which were picked up later by the researcher, providing an opportunity for personal contact, questions or screening for missing data. Some outpatients were in a hurry or under some other pressure (e.g., left glasses at home) and preferred to take the questionnaire with them and send it back in a prepared (stamped addressed) envelope. The researcher or ward physician collected the biomedical data. In many situations, however, it was necessary to wait for the results of examinations, because tumor activity and stage were unclear at the time of the research intervention.

Data Analysis

Data were transferred from written documents to a database file (Filemaker). Statistical analyses were performed with technical and intellectual support from the statistical unit and the Quality of Life Office of the Swiss Institute for Applied Cancer Research in Bern, using SAS and S-plus.

Descriptive statistics were used to classify data and to give information about the characteristics of the study population. Inferential statistics were used to identify the significance of differences in fatigue, anxiety and depression between different groups of the study population. Significance testing was performed by applying the Kruskal-Wallis test to the comparison of fatigue, anxiety and depression between patients with different types and stages of cancer and by further examining influencing factors, such as treatment, age and gender. Differences in proportions were tested with a chi-square test. For the three largest disease groups, fatigue was further analyzed by two-way ANOVA with the variables disease and stage, using type III error sums of scores (SAS Proc GLM). Correlation between results of different subscales of fatigue measurement, anxiety and depression was calculated with Pearson correlation coefficients.

Construct validity of the FAQ was examined by factor analysis after promax rotation. This method was used to ascertain the relationship between the variables measured and prior expectations on the basis of the underlying theory of the aspects investigated (De Vellis 1991), to further examine types of fatigue as defined in the previous chapter. Internal consistency of the FAQ as a whole and also its hypothesized physical, affective and cognitive subscales was examined using the Kudar Richardson 20 formula, a special form of coefficient alpha (for dichotomous answers). The internal consistency of the subscales was also examined with the Pearson correlation coefficients of the items within the subscales (for interval and ordinal scales, to test that correlation was different from zero). Correlation between all items of the whole questionnaire was analyzed with Pearson correlation coefficients.

Results

Characteristics of the Study Population

Of 682 consecutively asked cancer patients, 68 patients refused to participate in the study and 31 did not return the questionnaire, giving an overall response rate of 86% (Table 1). A further 71 patients were not able to fill in the questionnaire due to language and other problems as described in Table 1.

Table 1. Patient participation, response rate to, and acceptance and feasibility of the Fatigue Assessment Questionnaire (FAQ)

	Number of individuals involved			
	(*n*)	(%)	Subtotals	
			(*n*)	(%)
Patients eligible to participate in the study	682	100		
Reasons for patient nonparticipation:				
Patient refusal	68			
Questionnaire not returned	31			
Response rate			583	86
Further reasons for patient nonparticipation:				
Physically or psychologically unable to fill out questionnaire	23			
Cognitive impairment	11			
Language problems	33			
Selection error	4			
All participants			512	
Completed questionnaires	512			
Questionnaires not evaluable	13	3		
Evaluable questionnaires			499	97
Questionnaires completed at home		2		
Questionnaires completed in the treatment setting[a]		98		

[a] Participating institutions: Kantonsspital St. Gallen, Medizinische Klinik C 63% (316), Gynecology Department 7% (36), Radio-oncology Department 3% (16); Inselspital Bern, Institute of Oncology 16% (78), private oncology practice (Dr. Späti) 6% (31); Regionalspital Herisau, Oncology Department 5% (22).

Only 13 questionnaires from 512 patients were not able to be evaluated, which represents 97% evaluable questionnaires, of which 98% were completed in the hospital setting and 2% at home. Four hospitals with six departments were involved in the multi-institutional study. The final convenience sample consisted of 499 cancer patients.

Patient characteristics are presented in Table 2. Median age was 58 years for all participants and there was no major difference in age, with medians of 59 years in women and 56 years in men. Women outnumbered men by 61% to 39%. Most (82%) lived with others, only 12% living alone. Thirty-five percent of the whole study population were in full-time employment, and 15% worked part time. Eighteen percent were unable to work because of their illness, and 32% were retired.

Further disease characteristics of the patients are presented in Table 3. Of the 499 cancer patients, 51% suffered from metastatic and 14% from localized disease; 35% were living with disease in remission. Slightly more than half of the study population (58%) were undergoing cancer treatment at the

Table 2. Patient characteristics: I. Age, gender, social situation, employment ($n = 499$)

Characteristic	Median	Range	Percentage (%)
Age			
All (years)	58	18–91	
Women (years)	59	19–91	
Men (years)	56	18–86	
Gender			
Female			61
Male			39
Social situation			18
Living alone			82
Living with others			
Working			
Full-time			35
50%–99% of the time			10
1%–49% of the time			5
Unable to work			18
Retired			32

Table 3. Patient characteristics: II. Disease stage, treatment, Karnofsky Index, need for assistance in activities of daily living, and treatment setting ($n = 499$)

Characteristic	No. of patients	
	(n)	(%)
Cancer stage		
Localized	70	14
Metastatic	256	51
In remission	173	35
Cancer treatment		
Yes	291	58
No	208	42
Cancer treatment		
With active disease	217	78
With inactive disease	61	22
No cancer treatment		
With active disease	79	36
With inactive disease	138	64
Karnofsky Index		
100	212	42
80–99	248	50
51–79	35	7
<50	4	1
Need of assistance in activities of daily living[a]		
Yes	10	2
No	488[b]	98
Treatment setting		
Inpatient	94	19
Outpatient	405	81

[a] Patients self-assessed.
[b] Data unavailable in one case.

Table 4. Patient characteristics: III. Type and stage of cancer in percentages ($n=499$)

Type/stage of cancer	All ($n=499$; 100%)		Localized ($n=70$; 14%)	Metastatic ($n=256$; 51%)	In remission ($n=173$; 35%)
	(n)	(%)	(%)	(%)	(%)
Lung cancer	28	6	32	57	11
Breast cancer	149	30	13	41	46
Malignant lymphoma	115	23	10	60	30
Gastrointestinal cancers	64	13	6	66	28
Prostate cancer	11	2	10	72	18
Cancer of the testis	32	6	9	25	66
Ovarian cancer	19	5	19	62	19
Gynecological cancer (cervix, endometrium, vagina)	24	5	8	29	63
Melanoma	17	3	24	47	29
Others	33	7	33	61	6

Table 5. Patient characteristics: IV. Antineoplastic treatment within the last 2 months ($n=499$)

Treatment	Percentages (combinations not included) (%)	Percentages (combinations included) (%)
Chemotherapy	30.7	37.3
Hormone therapy	11.8	13.6
Immunotherapy	2.0	4.2
Radiotherapy	2.0	3.8
Combination therapy	7.8	–
Surgery	4.0	6.8
No treatment	41.7	41.7

time of the investigation. Forty-two percent of the whole study population had a Karnofsky Index of 100; an Index of 80–99 was observed in 50%, an Index of 60–79 in 7%, and only 1% had an Index of less than 50. This explained the low rate of self-assessed need of assistance in activities of daily living, which was reported by only 2% of the whole study population. Of the patients, 81% were treated on an outpatient basis, and the remaining 19% were hospitalized.

Table 4 presents the distribution of different types of cancer. The diagnosis was breast cancer in 30% of the patients, malignant lymphoma (including myeloma) in 23%, gastrointestinal cancer in 13%, lung cancer in 6%, cancer of the testis in 6%, ovarian cancer in 5%, gynecological cancer in 5%, malig-

Table 6. Patient characteristics: V. Regular use of other medications (non-antineoplastic) ($n=499$)

User/Nonuser	In percent (%)
Nonusers	48
Users	52
Type of Medication[a]	
Pain medication	14.8
Psychoactive drugs	5.8
Sleep medication	7.6
Others	37.9
Corticosteroids	3.0

[a] Some users use more than one medication.

nant melanoma in 3%, and "other" in 7%. The median time since diagnosis varied from 33 to 71 months.

The type of antineoplastic treatment involved is presented in Table 5. Of the patients, 30% underwent chemotherapy, 11% hormone therapy, 2% immunotherapy and 2% radiotherapy. Seven percent received a combined treatment. Forty-one percent of the patients had received no cancer treatment within the last 6 weeks. Approximately half of the study population (52%) received some other, non-cancer-specific medication (Table 6). In 37% this was medication for a medical condition other than cancer, such as cardiovascular disease, in 14% it was pain medication, in 7%, sleep medication, in 5%, psychoactive drugs, and 3% were receiving corticosteroids at the time of investigation.

Psychometric Properties of the FAQ

Content validity of FAQ was originally supported by the fact that the items of the instrument were derived from descriptors of fatigue, as identified in qualitative interviews by cancer patients themselves, who can be seen as experts in this respect (see report on preliminary study, chapter: "A Qualitative Exploration of the Concept of Fatigue/Tiredness in Cancer Patients and in Healthy Individuals"). Another earlier study testing the questionnaire in healthy individuals and in cancer patients supported content validity (see previous chapter).

Table 7 shows that all original FAQ items were reported by the whole study population and that again the items of the subscale "physical fatigue" were more frequently registered than the affective and cognitive items, which were used by under 30% of the patients. The percentage of reported items did vary in specific patient groups, which shows that the instrument is sensitive enough to detect differences. The replicated use of all items in this study supported the idea that they represented the content domain of fatigue.

Criterion-related validity was difficult to assess, as no comparable instrument was available in German and convergent validity therefore could not be

Table 7. Occurrence of fatigue in the overall patient population ($n=499$), measured with the items of the Fatigue Assessment Questionnaire (FAQ)

Ranking	Binary item (item number in FAQ)	Occurrence in percent (%)
1	Experiencing pleasant tiredness (14)	62
2	Decreased physical performance (16)	59
3	Loss of energy (20)	53
4	Weakness (19)	49
5	Fight to overcome inactivity (21)	45
6	Unusual need for rest (2)	44
7	Feeling sleepy during the day (23)	42
8	Wish to switch off thoughts (15)	41
9	Feeling unusually tired (6)	39
10	Becoming slower (1)	37
10	Sleep problems at night (3)	37
11	Feeling tense (11)	36
12	Having heavy limbs (13)	35
13	Wish to withdraw (4)	34
14	Decreased attentiveness (17)	33
15	Feeling impatient (18)	32
16	Increased forgetfulness (9)	28
16	Difficulties in concentrating (4)	28
17	Experiencing malaise (12)	25
18	Sadness (22)	24
19	Feeling exhausted (7)	23
20	Loss of interest (19)	19
21	Anxiety (8)	18

tested directly. The different stages of cancer, which were hypothesized to correlate with fatigue, however, can be used as an external criterion. As the instrument was able to assess differences between the different stages of cancer (see Tables 13, 14), which can be seen as support for criterion-related validity, this could also be seen as a type of known group validation. Validity concerning feasibility and acceptability was established by the high rate of correctly completed questionnaires (97%). The response rate of 86% also supported the important aspect of face validity.

Construct validity was examined using factor analytic techniques (promax rotation). Factor loadings are presented in Table 8. Three factors could be established, supporting the hypothesis proposed earlier of a theoretical framework of fatigue as a multidimensional construct, with expression at physical,

Table 8. Factor loadings after promax rotation of the FAQ and eigenvalue of the items ($n=465$)

Questionnaire items	Factor 1, physical	Factor 2, affective	Factor 3, cognitive	Eigenvalue
1 Becoming slower	**0.73**[a]	0.02	0.06	7.4958
2 Unusual need for rest	**0.90**	0.00	0.01	1.9241
3 Sleep problems at night	0.01	0.70	0.12	1.3984
4 Difficulties in concentrating	0.02	0.01	**0.91**	1.1149
5 Wish to withdraw	0.31	0.42	0.01	1.0221
6 Feeling unusually tired	**0.91**	0.01	0.01	0.9577
7 Feeling exhausted	0.41	0.36	0.00	0.9156
8 Anxiety	0.00	**1.00**	−0.03	0.7962
9 Increased forgetfulness	0.02	0.00	**1.00**	0.7666
10 Weakness	**1.00**	0.00	0.00	0.6884
11 Feeling tense	0.02	**0.85**	0.02	0.6503
12 Feeling unwell	**0.62**	0.15	0.00	0.6112
13 Having heavy limbs	**0.94**	0.02	0.00	0.6051
14 Experiencing pleasant tiredness	−0.51	0.00	0.25	0.5879
15 Wish to switch off thoughts	0.00	**0.88**	0.07	0.5379
16 Decreased physical performance	**0.94**	0.00	0.02	0.5254
17 Decreased attentiveness	0.03	0.01	**0.89**	0.4541
18 Feeling impatient	0.00	**0.88**	0.07	0.4398
19 Loss of interest	0.56	0.23	0.00	0.3950
20 Loss of energy	**0.93**	0.00	0.01	0.3637
21 Fight to overcome inactivity	**0.78**	0.01	0.05	0.2792
22 Sadness	0.02	**0.97**	−0.05	0.2621
23 Feeling sleepy during the day	**0.52**	0.01	0.21	0.2086

[a] Loadings printed in bold indicate to what subscale the items were aggregated, considering the value of loading and the researcher's professional judgment.

affective and cognitive levels (see the chapters "A Qualitative Exploration of the Concept of Fatigue/Tiredness in Cancer Patients and in Healthy Individuals," and "Testing the Fatigue Assessment Questionnaire in Healthy Persons and in Cancer Patients"). Factor analysis showed that the items "wish to withdraw," "feeling exhausted," "loss of interest" and "pleasant tiredness" were not related to any factor and these were therefore deleted from the instrument before data analyses began. The instrument now comprised 19 binary items and a physical (11 items), an affective (5 items) and a cognitive (3 items) subscale, as well as a fourth single-item scale involving "sleep problems," and LASA scales to measure quantity and distress of fatigue. The item "sleeping problems at night" (identified in the qualitative interviews), showing no relation to the three identified factors, was used as a single-item scale

Table 9. Subscales of the FAQ identified by factor analysis after promax rotation and correlation of items with subscales[a] ($n=465$). Overall reliability of the entire scale: 0.90 (correlation alpha, Kudar Richardson formula 20)

Subscale/subscale item	Coefficient
Overall reliability of the entire scale: $r=0.90$	
Physical fatigue subscale ($r=0.90$)[a]	
Becoming slower	0.64
Unusual need for rest	0.74
Feeling unusually tired	0.73
Feeling exhausted	0.51
Weakness	0.79
Feeling unwell	0.49
Having heavy limbs	0.43
Decreased physical performance	0.69
Loss of energy	0.73
Fight to overcome inactivity	0.70
Feeling sleepy during the day	0.53
Cognitive fatigue subscale ($r=0.68$)[a]	
Difficulties in concentrating	0.54
Increased forgetfulness	0.43
Decreased attentiveness	0.50
Affective fatigue subscale ($r=0.65$)[a]	
Anxiety	0.43
Feeling tense	0.44
Wish to switch off thoughts	0.34
Feeling impatient	0.33
Sadness	0.49
Single item subscale	
Sleeping problems at night	

The items "wish to withdraw," "experiencing pleasant tiredness," and "loss of interest" were deleted due to difficulty in assigning them to a factor.
[a] Pearson correlation between the single item and the subscale, reduced by this item.

because it was hypothesized that it was a separate concept with an influence on a possible activity/inactivity imbalance (see the chapter "A Qualitative Exploration of the Concept of Fatigue/Tiredness in Cancer Patients and in Healthy Individuals"). The adapted FAQ is presented in the Appendix 1.

To search for support of the reliability of the FAQ, internal consistency was examined. A special version of the alpha coefficient (the Kuder-Richardson formula 20, for dichotomous items) was calculated after the identification of subscales by factor analyses and after deletion of redundant items. The reliability coefficient was then 0.90 for the overall scale, 0.90 for the physical subscale, 0.65 for the affective subscale and 0.68 for the cognitive subscale. The correlation coefficients (Pearson) of the items within the subscales supported the three-factor solution (Table 9).

It was difficult to establish stability (one element of reliability), as a test-retest was not appropriate for measuring a fluctuating construct like fatigue.

Table 10. Types of cancer and fatigue, measured with the FAQ subscales ($n=499$)

Type of cancer	Fatigue (FAQ) subscales "Last week"						
	Physical		Affective		Cognitive		Sleeping problems
	Mean	SD	Mean	SD	Mean	SD	(%)
Lung cancer (28)	7.0	3.1	1.9	1.4	1.3	1.0	68
Breast cancer (149)	3.8	3.6	1.4	1.4	0.8	1.0	36
Malignant lymphoma (115)	4.5	3.6	1.4	1.5	0.8	1.1	31
Gastrointestinal cancers (64)	4.4	3.7	1.1	1.1	0.6	0.9	37
Prostate cancer (11)	4.9	3.8	1.2	1.2	1.1	1.1	27
Cancer of the testis (32)	3.6	4.1	2.0	1.5	0.8	1.0	41
Ovarian cancer (26)	5.4	3.6	1.1	1.2	0.8	0.9	31
Gynecological cancer (endometrium, cervix, vagina) (24)	2.5	4.1	1.6	1.4	0.9	1.0	46
Melanoma (17)	5.5	3.9	1.8	1.3	1.2	1.1	29
Others (33)	5.5	3.7	2.0	1.7	1.1	1.2	45
p values (Kruskal-Wallis test)	0.005		0.03		0.13		

Stability, however, could be supported by reproducibility of consistent results with the FAQ subscales and the FAQ LASA scales in different stages of cancer (see Tables 13, 14 and accompanying text).

Correlation of Fatigue with Different Types of Cancer

Table 10 shows a statistical difference in physical fatigue between all cancer types ($p=0.005$). A less significant difference in affective fatigue was also established between all cancer types ($p=0.03$), but no difference was found for cognitive fatigue ($p=0.13$). Patients with cancer of the lung, prostate, or ovaries and the groups with melanoma and mixed cancer types showed the most prominent difference between physical and affective fatigue.

Table 11 shows the results of quantitative levels of fatigue in the different types of cancer, as measured with the LASA (Linear Analogue Scale Assessment) scales of FAQ. Even though a difference in fatigue levels between the different types of cancer can be observed, these differences are not statistically significant, apart from a trend for significance for the measurement period of last month ($p=0.06$) and for the period of the last six months ($p=0.08$). Levels of fatigue were, however, highest ranked in patients with lung and ovarian cancer for the period of last week and last month. Patients with breast and gastrointestinal cancer showed stable fatigue levels over the three measurement periods, whereas lung cancer showed an increase from the last six months towards last week. Fatigue distress, as measured with the

Table 11. Type of cancer, fatigue and fatigue distress, measured with the LASA (Linear Analogue Scale Assessment) scales of FAQ ($n=499$)

Type of Cancer	Fatigue "last week"		Fatigue "last month"		Fatigue in last six months		Fatigue distress	
	Mean	SD	Mean	SD	Mean	SD	Mean	SD
Lung cancer	50.1	25.0	47.1	24.1	40.5	25.6	42.6	28.0
Breast cancer	34.2	28.6	32.3	26.4	31.6	27.3	33.0	29.3
Malignant lymphoma	33.3	26.2	38.4	28.3	36.0	28.8	35.2	29.3
Gastrointestinal cancers	36.2	27.4	36.5	27.7	33.0	25.9	38.3	29.7
Prostate cancer	38.0	23.5	39.2	20.2	43.6	21.6	38.2	27.9
Cancer of the testis	28.7	28.8	26.4	26.0	25.2	24.8	7.3	27.4
Ovarian cancer	45.5	32.8	47.3	31.8	46.0	23.9	40.3	34.7
Gynecological cancer (endometrium, cervix, vagina)	35.0	30.2	31.6	28.8	27.1	30.3	24.3	34.7
Melanoma	37.7	30.6	37.5	24.9	35.4	24.0	24.2	20.1
Others	36.9	27.4	38.8	26.8	33.8	29.1	32.1	29.5
p (Kruskal-Wallis test)	0.17		0.06		0.08		0.18	

LASA scale of FAQ, is also presented in Table 11. Again, no statistically significant difference was found between any of the types of cancer ($p=0.18$). However, the fatigue distress levels were ranked highest in association with lung and ovarian cancer, followed by prostate cancer, melanoma and gastrointestinal cancer. To illustrate these differences better, fatigue levels for last week, last month and fatigue distress (measured with LASA scales of FAQ) in the groups with different cancer types are presented as box plots in Figs. 1 and 2. Physical, affective and cognitive fatigue (measured with the subscales with dichotomous items of FAQ) in the groups with different types of cancer are presented as box plots in the Figs. 2 and 3.

Analyzing Fatigue in the Different Stages of Breast Cancer, Malignant Lymphoma and Gastrointestinal Cancers

The three largest patient groups, with breast cancer, malignant lymphoma and gastrointestinal cancer, were further analyzed (Table 12, see p. 128)).

In patients with breast cancer, a significant difference in physical fatigue (FAQ physical subscale) was found, the highest physical fatigue levels being reported by those with localized disease, followed by metastatic disease, followed by disease in remission ($p=0.001$). This was not the case for affective fatigue measured by the FAQ affective subscale ($p=0.38$) or for cognitive fatigue measured by the FAQ cognitive subscale ($p=0.15$). No significant dif-

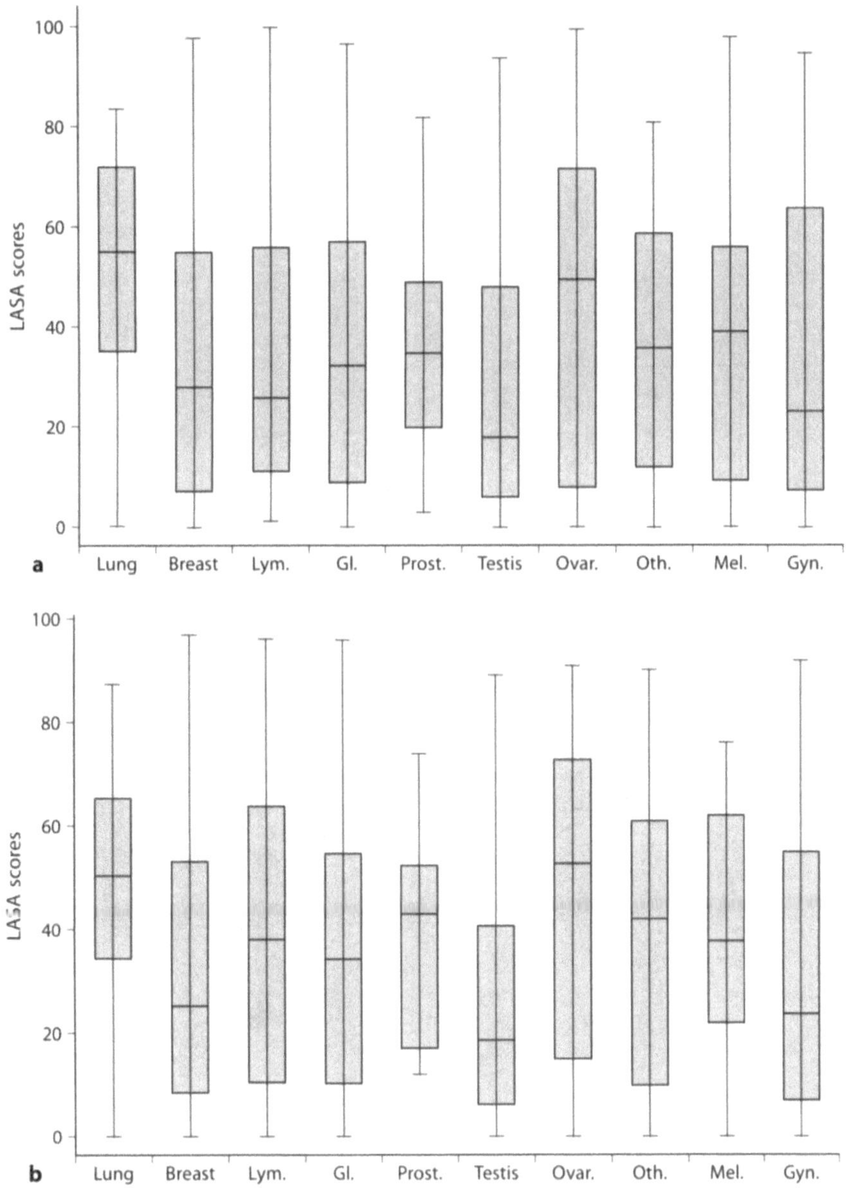

Fig. 1. Fatigue levels in different types of cancer **a** last week and **b** last month. *LYM.*, lymphoma; *GI.*, gastrointestinal; *PROST.*, prostate; *OVAR.*, ovarian; *OTH.*, other; *MEL.*, melanoma; *GYN.*, gynecological

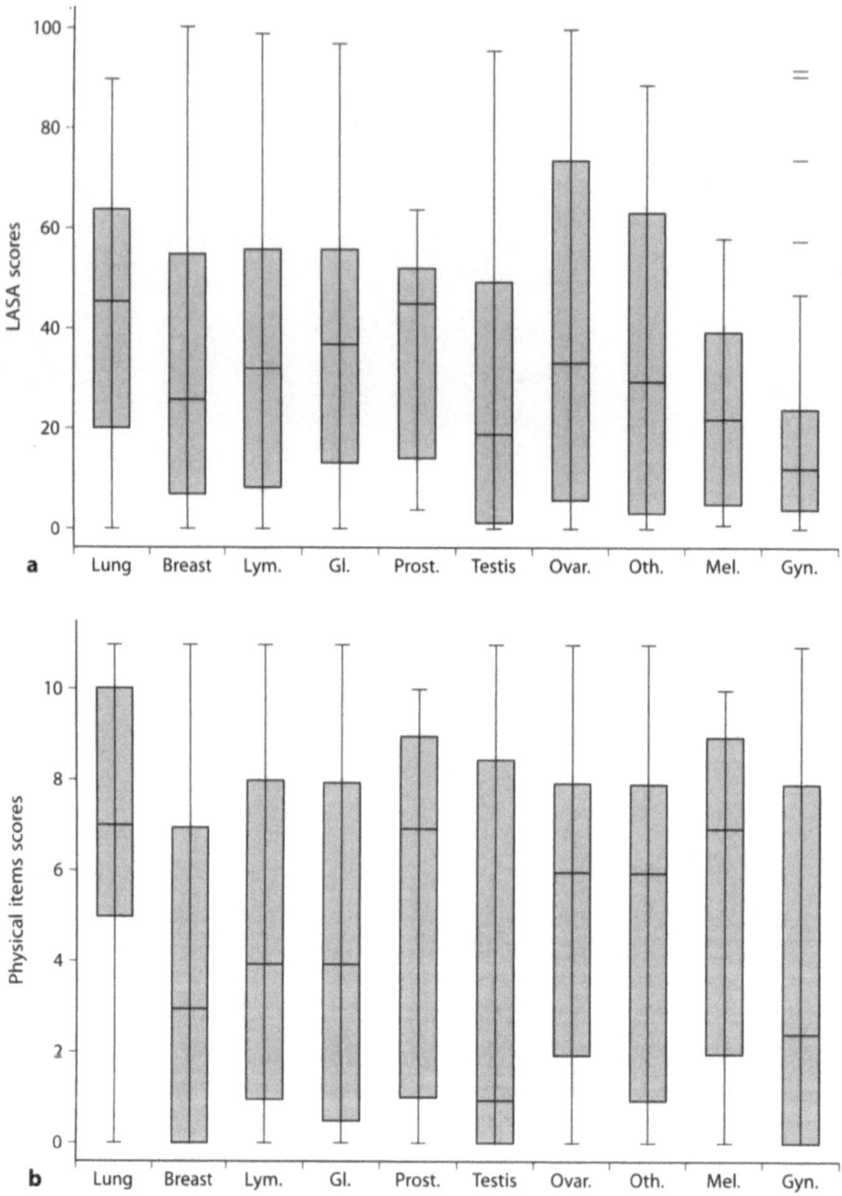

Fig. 2. a Levels of distress caused by fatigue in different types of cancer. **b** Physical fatigue in different types of cancer

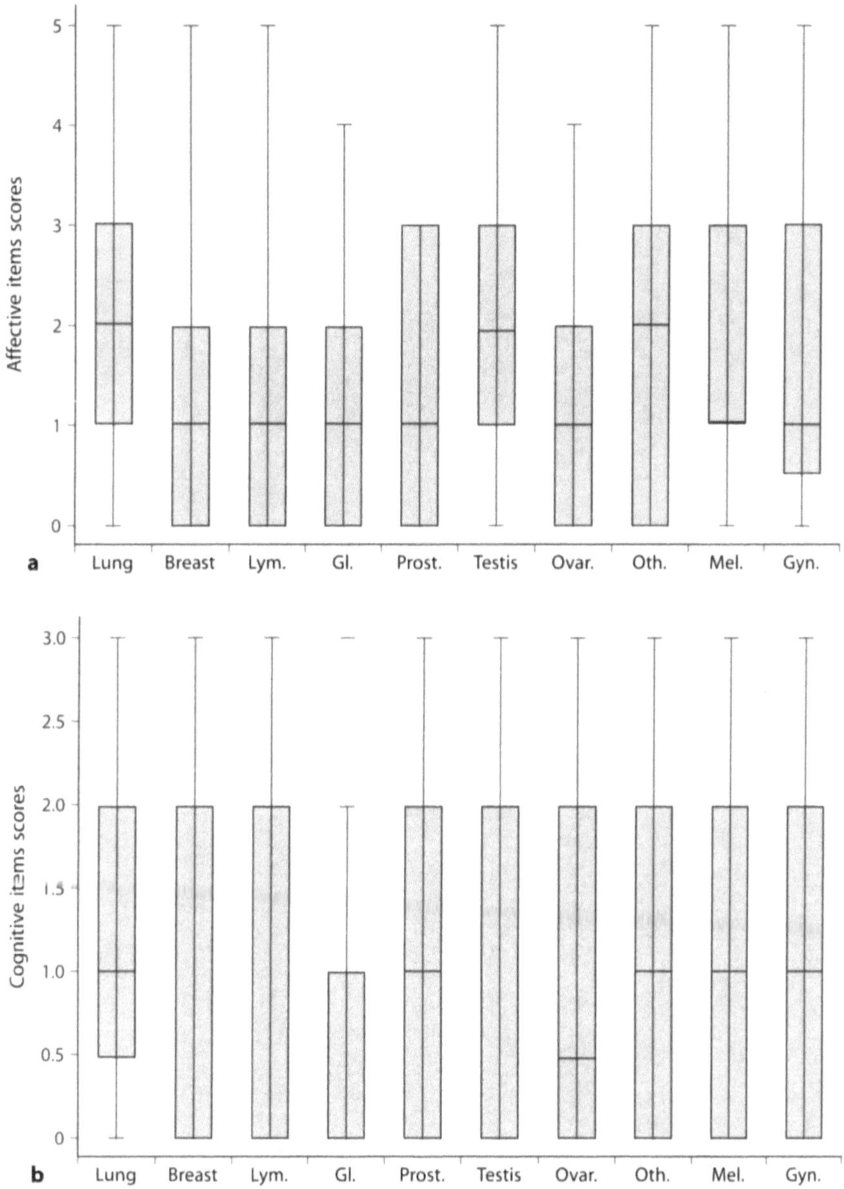

Fig. 3. a Affective and **b** cognitive fatigue in different types of cancer

Table 12. Differences between breast cancer, malignant lymphoma and gastrointestinal cancers in relation to fatigue subscales, fatigue intensity and its distress as measured with the FAQ subscales, FAQ LASA scales and with the Hospital Anxiety and Depression Scales

Type of cancer	Fatigue last week						Fatigue last week		Fatigue last month		Fatigue last 6 months		Fatigue distress		Sleep problems	HADS-A		HADS-D	
	Physical		Affective		Cognitive		LASA		LASA		LASA		LASA		(%)				
	Mean	SD	Mean	SD	Mean	SD	Mean	SD	Mean	SD	Mean	SD	Mean	SD		Mean	SD	Mean	SD
Breast cancer ($n=149$)																			
In remission (68)	2.7	3.2	1.3	1.4	0.6	1.0	27.9	26.9	27.1	26.9	26.0	26.8	28.7	28.8	41	4.5	3.0	2.6	2.5
Localized disease (19)	5.4	3.9	1.5	1.4	0.8	1.1	38.7	30.2	39.3	25.7	35.5	28.2	44.0	32.5	47	6.9	4.3	4.7	3.5
Metastatic disease (62)	4.5	3.7	1.5	1.4	1.0	1.0	39.8	28.9	35.9	25.8	36.6	27.0	34.8	28.4	25	5.2	3.3	4.1	3.4
p^a	0.001		0.38		0.15		0.37		0.48		0.06		0.14		0.09	0.08		0.005	
Malignant lymphoma ($n=115$)																			
In remission (34)	2.3	7.4	0.9	1.1	0.5	(0.8)	22.7	21.7	23.0	23.4	22.2	21.6	29.2	21.1	20	3.5	2.8	2.5	2.7
Localized disease (12)	4.8	3.2	1.8	1.7	1.0	(1.3)	34.6	30.2	36.0	29.8	26.8	26.4	32.0	32.1	50	5.8	3.5	4.8	2.7
Metastatic disease (69)	5.5	3.5	1.5	1.6	0.9	(1.1)	38.2	26.4	46.4	27.4	44.5	29.5	43.6	29.3	33	5.7	3.7	4.9	3.6
p^a	0.001		0.07		0.22		0.01		0.0002		0.0008		0.0003		0.14	0.005		0.0004	
Gastrointestinal cancers ($n=64$)																			
In remission (18)	3.3	3.5	0.7	1.1	0.8	1.0	30.1	28.5	33.7	30.5	37.3	28.6	32.6	27.3	44	4.2	3.2	3.3	3.6
Localized disease (4)	1.2	2.5	1.5	1.7	0.5	1.0	28.5	45.7	29.5	44.6	18.0	13.4	31.0	44.6	25	4.7	2.9	1.5	1.2
Metastatic disease (42)	5.2	3.6	1.2	1.0	0.6	0.9	39.5	25.1	38.3	25.3	32.1	25.4	41.6	26.6	35	5.4	3.0	5.1	3.3
p^b	0.07		0.08		0.45		0.17		0.40		0.61		0.36		0.52	0.21		0.03	

HADS-A, Hospital Anxiety and Depression Scales, Anxiety; HADS-D, Hospital Anxiety and Depression Scales, Depression
[a] Kruskal-Wallis test
[b] Wilcoxon two-sample test (in remission versus all others)

ference was found either for the quantity of fatigue (LASA) for the three time periods of measurement, or for the distress it caused. A trend was found for all measures to be higher in breast cancer patients with localized disease than in those with metastatic disease. Looking at anxiety, mean results varied between 4.5 and 6.9, not reaching any significant difference. Depression, however, differed significantly between the three stages ($p=0.005$), with higher levels in breast cancer patients with localized disease, followed by metastatic disease.

In patients with malignant lymphoma, a significant difference was again found in physical fatigue, with highest levels in patients with metastatic disease, followed by localized disease and disease in remission ($p=0.001$). This was not the case for affective fatigue ($p=0.07$) and cognitive fatigue ($p=0.22$). A significant difference was found for the quantity of fatigue (LASA) for last week ($p=0.01$) and an even more robust difference for the period of last month ($p=0.0002$) and for the last six months ($p=0.0003$). Sleep problems, although not significantly different, were also more prominent in lymphoma patients with localized disease than in those with metastatic disease. Looking at anxiety, a significant difference was found between the stages of lymphoma with highest levels in *metastatic* disease, followed by localized disease and disease in remission ($p=0.005$). The same was the case for depression ($p=0.0004$).

In patients with gastrointestinal cancer, no statistical difference was detected between disease in remission and localized plus metastatic disease (as one group), apart from the levels of depression (0.03), which were higher in metastatic disease than in localized disease or disease in remission.

When the three groups of patients with breast cancer, malignant lymphoma and gastrointestinal cancer were compared using two-way ANOVA with stage as the second factor, no statistical difference was found between the three diagnoses. The other types of cancer were not further analyzed because of the relatively small numbers.

Correlation of Fatigue with Different Stages of Cancer

The association of fatigue with different stages of all cancer types was found to be statistically significant (Table 13). The association with physical fatigue, as measured with the physical subscale of the FAQ, was highly significant, with highest levels in metastatic disease, followed by localized disease and disease in remission (0.0001).

The association with affective fatigue remained significant (0.02), although less significant than the association with physical fatigue, and the same was the case for cognitive fatigue (0.03). No difference was found between stages in cancer and sleeping problems ($p=0.76$). The association of fatigue with stages of cancer was statistically significant when measured with the LASA scale of FAQ (Table 14) for the periods of last week ($p=0.0001$), last month ($p=0.0001$) and last six months ($p=0.0002$). Whereas mean levels of fatigue

Table 13. Stage of cancer and fatigue, measured with the FAQ subscales, HADS and the Karnofsky Index ($n=499$)

	Fatigue						Sleeping Problems	HADS-A		HADS-D		Karnofsky Index
	Physical		Affective		Cognitive							
	Mean	SD	Mean	SD	Mean	SD	(%)	Mean	SD	Mean	SD	Mean
Stage of cancer												
In remission (173)	3.0	3.3	1.2	1.4	0.7	1.0	37%	4.3	3.2	2.7	2.8	100
Localized disease (70)	4.0	3.9	1.7	1.5	0.9	1.1	41%	5.7	3.7	4.2	3.1	90
Metastatic disease (256)	5.4	3.6	1.5	1.4	0.9	1.0	37%	5.5	3.5	4.9	3.5	90
p (Kruskal-Wallis test)	0.0001		0.02		0.03		0.76	0.0004		0.0001		

Table 14. Fatigue and fatigue distress, measured with the LASA scales of FAQ, according to stage of cancer ($n=499$)

	Fatigue						Fatigue distress	
	Last week		Last month		Last 6 months			
	Mean	SD	Mean	SD	Mean	SD	Mean	SD
Stage of cancer								
In remission	28.9	26.5	28.4	28.4	28.2	26.2	27.2	26.7
Localized disease	35.4	29.9	34.0	28.2	29.7	26.9	33.5	31.2
Metastatic disease	40.5	27.7	42.1	26.8	38.9	27.3	39.0	28.8
p (Kruskal-Wallis test)	0.0001		0.0001		0.0002		0.002	

remained stable from last six months to last week in patients with disease in remission, fatigue levels showed a tendency to increase in patients with metastatic disease and localized disease from the last six months towards the last week period. Fatigue distress was also found to be significantly different between the stages ($p=0.0002$), as measured with the LASA scale of FAQ, with the highest levels in metastatic disease, followed by localized disease and disease in remission. The mean levels for fatigue and for fatigue distress were approximately the same, which emphasizes its relevance.

Influence of Anticancer Treatment on Fatigue in All Patients

Table 15 presents the mean fatigue levels, measured with the LASA scale of FAQ, for last week and last month in relation to the different treatment modalities (in millimeters). Immunotherapy (only ten patients) was associated with the highest levels of fatigue (51), followed by chemotherapy (42), and then by radiotherapy (40; only six patients). Mean levels of fatigue were lower for the patients receiving hormone therapy (29) and after surgery within the last 6 weeks (34) than with the other treatment regimens. The mean levels of fatigue in patients receiving any kind of anticancer treatment was 38, while the mean levels of those receiving no cancer treatment at all was 31.

Examination of fatigue levels in all patients receiving anticancer treatment and comparison of them with those in patients who did not (Table 16) revealed statistically significantly higher levels in the treated group (LASA scale of FAQ) for last week (0.005) and last month (0.003), and also more fatigue distress (0.002). Patients with antineoplastic treatment also reported statistically significantly more physical fatigue (FAQ subscale) than those without anticancer treatment (0.0001), whereas no significant difference was found for affective fatigue (0.62) or cognitive fatigue (0.56). Sleeping problems did not differ between the two groups ($p=0.58$).

Table 15. Differences in fatigue intensity in relation to different types of treatment, measured with the LASA scales of FAQ ($n=499$)

	Fatigue (FAQ LASA) (mm)			
	Last week		Last month	
	Mean	SD	Mean	SD
Chemotherapy, all ($n=153$)	42.0	28.5	43.3	26.5
Without noncancer medications (55)	37.2	26.4	42.4	26.7
With noncancer medications (98)	46.2	29.3	43.9	26.6
Hormone therapy, all ($n=59$)	29.0	25.5	30.5	26.0
Without noncancer medications (22)	25.2	25.1	28.4	25.4
With noncancer medications (37)	31.3	25.8	31.8	26.7
Immunotherapy, all (n=10)	51.2	32.5	58.7	27.8
Without noncancer medications (3)	56.6	17.2	54.6	21.0
With noncancer medications (7)	48.8	38.3	60.4	31.6
Radiotherapy, all ($n=6$)	40.2	34.0	43.2	36.9
Without noncancer medications				
With noncancer medication (6)	45.8	33.6	49.3	36.4
Combination therapy ($n=39$)	34.8	25.2	35.5	24.6
Without noncancer medications (12)	33.3	25.6	39.2	24.5
With noncancer medications (27)	35.5	26.1	33.9	24.9
Surgery, all ($n=29$)	34.7	25.5	30.9	31.1
Without noncancer medications (12)	32.7	25.9	19.5	25.3
With noncancer medications (8)	37.6	26.3	48.0	32.6
No cancer treatment, all ($n=207$)	31.8	27.7	32.0	26.9
Without noncancer medications	29.0	27.7	30.3	27.6
With noncancer medications	36.8	27.2	34.9	25.4
All cancer treatment (n=291)	38.6	28.0	39.3	27.4
Without noncancer medication	*31.0*	*27.0*	*27.0*	*33.0*
With noncancer medication	*40.0*	*28.4*	*39.2*	*27.4*
p (Kruskal-Wallis test)	0.0004		0.003	

Influence of Anticancer Treatment on Fatigue in Patients with Different Stages of Cancer

In patients with cancer in remission, no difference was found between those with and without anticancer medication in any of the three stages. In patients with localized disease, a difference between the groups with and without anticancer treatment in the different stages of cancer was found only in physical fatigue (physical fatigue subscale), together with a slight, but nonsignificant difference in fatigue distress. In metastatic disease, no influence of the anticancer treatment was observed.

Table 16. Differences in treatment status in relation to fatigue and fatigue distress, measured with the LASA scales and subscales of FAQ and HADS ($n=499$)

Treatment status	Fatigue				Fatigue distress		FAQ subscales						Sleep Problems	HADS-A		HADS-D	
	Last week		Last month				Physical		Affective		Cognitive						
	Mean	SD	Mean	SD	Mean	SD	Mean	SD	Mean	SD	Mean	SD	%	Mean	SD	Mean	SD
Antineoplastic treatment																	
Yes (58%)	38	28.0	39	27.4	37	28.4	5.4	3.7	1.5	1.4	0.9	1.1	38%	5.3	3.4	4.3	3.4
No (42%)	31	27.7	32	26.9	30	29.2	3.6	3.6	1.5	1.5	0.7	1.0	36%	4.9	3.5	3.6	3.3
p^a	0.005		0.003		0.002		0.0001		0.62		0.56		0.58	0.08		0.004	
Non-cancer treatment																	
Yes (52%)	40	28.4	39.2	27.1	37.6	28.6	5.2	3.7	1.5	1.4	1.0	1.1	43%	5.5	3.7	4.6	3.6
No (48%)	31	27.0	33.0	27.4	30.4	28.8	3.7	3.6	1.4	1.4	0.7	1.0	32%	4.7	3.2	3.4	3.0
p^a	0.0004		0.007		0.001		0.0001		0.59		0.0001		0.009[b]	0.03		0.0001	

[a] Kruskal-Wallis test.
[b] Chi-square test.

Influence of Non-Anticancer Medications on Fatigue

Fatigue levels of the patients who received other medications than anticancer treatment (listed in Table 6), were different from those patients who did not need such medications. Table 16 shows the difference in fatigue between the patients receiving additional noncancer medication and those who did not receive any. Statistical analysis showed significantly higher fatigue levels in patients with additional noncancer medication (LASA of FAQ) for last week ($p=0.0004$) and last month ($p=0.007$) and with fatigue distress ($p=0.001$). Patients with additional noncancer medication also showed more physical fatigue ($p=0.001$) and cognitive fatigue ($p=0.0001$), whereas affective fatigue did not differ between the two groups ($p=0.59$). Those patients who received non-anti-cancer medication had more sleeping problems than the others ($p=0.009$).

Influence of Age and Gender on Fatigue in Cancer Patients

Table 17 presents differences in fatigue between age and gender. Comparison between patients younger than 50 years and patients older than 50 years showed that younger patients experienced more affective fatigue (affective subscale) than the older group ($p=0.02$). A trend could be observed towards more physical fatigue (physical subscale) ($p=0.06$) and fatigue distress as measured with LASA in the older patient group ($p=0.09$). Higher scores for depression were also observed in the older patient group ($p=0.005$).

The influence of gender on fatigue was not relevant when the whole study population was examined (Table 17). However, a difference was observed in depression scores between male and female patients: men presented higher scores for depression ($p=0.02$).

The investigation of fatigue and gender in different age groups showed that there was no difference between women under 50 years of age and women over 50 (Table 17). This was not the case in male patients: the group of men aged over 50 years showed significantly more physical fatigue ($p=0.005$) and also higher depression scores than those aged under 50 years ($p=0.001$).

Differences in Anxiety and Depression at Different Stages and with Different Types of Cancer, Karnofsky Index Scores and Types of Cancer Treatment

Table 18 presents the results obtained by measuring anxiety and depression with the Hospital Anxiety and Depression Scales (HADS). The overall mean of the anxiety scale showed a significant difference between the groups with highest anxiety scores in patients with localized disease, followed by patients with metastatic disease and then by those with disease in remission ($p=0.0004$). Anxiety items with highest mean scores were "anxious presenti-

Table 17. Variation in fatigue subscales, fatigue intensity and its distress as measured with the FAQ and HADS ($n=499$) according to age and gender

	Fatigue						Fatigue						Fatigue distress		HADS-A		HADS-D	
	Last week						Last week		Last month		Last 6 months							
	Physical		Affective		Cognitive		LASA		LASA		LASA		LASA					
	Mean	SD	Mean	SD	Mean	SD	Mean	SD	Mean	SD	Mean	SD	Mean	SD	Mean	SD	Mean	SD
Age																		
Under 50 years of age ($n=166$)	4.0	3.6	1.6	1.4	0.8	1.0	34.1	28.6	33.4	27.3	31.8	27.9	31.2	28.1	5.2	3.4	3.4	2.9
Over 50 years of age ($n=333$)	4.7	3.7	1.4	1.4	0.9	1.0	36.6	27.8	37.6	27.4	34.9	27.0	35.6	29.3	5.1	3.5	4.3	3.5
p^a	0.06		0.02		0.32		0.29		0.09		0.13		0.09		0.77		0.005	
Gender																		
Female ($n=306$)	4.3	3.7	1.4	1.5	0.9	1.0	36.8	29.1	36.2	28.1	35.1	28.1	35.4	30.2	5.1	3.5	3.8	3.3
Males($n=193$)	4.7	3.7	1.5	1.4	0.9	1.0	34.1	26.4	36.3	26.3	32.0	26.0	32.3	26.9	5.2	3.4	4.4	3.5
p^a	0.19		0.31		0.9[illegible]		0.49		0.90		0.28		0.35		0.75		0.02	
Females																		
Under 50 years of age	4.2	3.8	1.6	1.4	0.9	1.0	37.1	30.1	35.1	28.5	35.7	29.9	34.5	31.4	5.3	3.1	3.2	3.0
Over 50 years of age	4.3	3.4	1.4	1.5	0.9	1.0	36.7	28.7	36.6	28.1	34.9	27.5	35.7	29.8	5.0	3.4	3.9	3.4
p^a	0.71		0.15		0.99		0.93		0.63		0.91		0.54		0.57		0.11	
Males																		
Under 50 years of age	3.9	3.5	1.7	1.3	0.7	1.0	31.2	26.9	31.6	26.1	28.0	25.4	28.0	24.1	5.0	3.1	3.5	2.9
Over 50 years of age	5.4	3.6	14	1.4	0.9	1.0	36.4	25.9	39.8	26.0	35.1	26.1	35.6	28.4	5.3	3.6	5.2	3.7
p^a	0.005		0.13		0.[illegible]3		0.52		0.21		0.18		0.08		0.80		0.001	

[a] Wilcoxon two-sample test.

Table 18. Variations in the Hospital Anxiety and Depression Scale (HADS, German version) measuring anxiety and depression according to stage of cancer ($n=499$)

Items (translated from German into English)	Mean values and SDs as related to cancer stage						
	Localized		Metastatic		In remission		p^a
A1 Tension/irritation	0.84	0.69	0.92	0.74	0.77	0.68	0.09
A2 Anxious presentiments	1.21	0.93	1.09	0.87	0.73	0.82	0.0001
A3 Worrying thoughts	0.89	0.78	0.89	0.80	0.60	0.75	0.0002
A4 Ability to relax	0.72	0.74	0.68	0.74	0.56	0.65	0.21
A5 Anxious feeling in the stomach	0.64	0.72	0.66	0.65	0.54	0.64	0.13
A6 Restlessness	1.01	0.93	0.89	0.87	0.82	0.91	0.28
A7 Panic attacks	0.42	0.67	0.43	0.61	0.28	0.52	0.03
Mean for the anxiety subscale	*5.75*	*3.75*	*5.59*	*3.51*	*4.34*	*3.28*	*0.0004*
D1 Ability to enjoy as before	0.57	0.64	0.65	0.68	0.41	0.61	0.0007
D2 Laughing and seeing funny things	0.60	0.66	0.69	0.73	0.32	0.52	0.0001
D3 Happiness	0.41	0.71	0.56	0.75	0.29	0.56	0.0004
D4 Feeling held back	1.12	0.75	1.30	0.80	0.74	0.66	0.0001
D5 Loss of interest in appearance	0.38	0.72	0.39	0.69	0.18	0.50	0.001
D6 Enjoy future	0.78	0.81	0.96	0.83	0.56	0.73	0.0001
D7 Enjoying a book, radio, television	0.31	0.62	0.33	0.62	0.21	0.46	0.18
Mean for the depression subscale	*4.25*	*3.12*	*4.91*	*3.59*	*2.75*	*2.84*	*0.0001*

[a] Kruskal-Wallis test.

ments," "tension," and "worrying thoughts." All anxiety items showed lower scores in those cancer patients who were in remission.

The overall mean of the depression scale showed an even more significant difference between the groups, with the highest scores for depression in patients with metastatic disease, followed by patients with localized disease and then by patients with disease in remission ($p=0.0001$). Depression items with the highest mean scores were "feeling held back," "(not) enjoying future" and "(not) laughing and seeing funny things." All depression items showed lower scores in cancer patients in remission than in those with localized or metastatic disease.

Table 19 presents the different types of cancer and the related mean scores for anxiety and depression. Highest scores for anxiety and depression were observed in patients with lung cancer. Lowest anxiety scores were found in patients with prostate cancer (only 11 patients), and lowest depression scores in patients with cancer of the testicles. A significant difference was found for depression when all types of cancer were compared ($p=0.003$). This was not the case for anxiety ($p=0.53$). No difference was observed for anxiety or depression and the scores on the Karnofsky Index in all types of cancer together.

Table 19. Variation in mean values and SD for anxiety and depression (HADS) and in median for Karnofsky Index according to type of cancer ($n=499$)

Type of cancer	No. of patients	HADS-A		HADS-D		Karnofsky Index
		Mean	SD	Mean	SD	Median
Lung cancer	28	6.6	3.8	6.0	3.3	80
Breast cancer	149	5.1	3.3	3.5	3.1	90
Malignant lymphoma	115	5.1	3.6	4.1	3.4	90
Gastrointestinal cancers	64	5.0	3.0	4.3	3.4	90
Prostate cancer	11	3.6	2.0	4.3	4.7	90
Cancer of the testis	32	5.0	3.3	2.5	2.2	100
Ovarian cancer	26	5.0	5.5	4.3	3.3	90
Gynecological cancer (endometrium, cervix, vagina)	24	5.0	4.9	3.8	4.2	100
Melanoma	17	5.1	3.0	4.7	2.7	90
Others	33	5.3	3.6	4.6	3.8	90
p (Kruskal-Wallis test)		0.53		0.003		

Table 20. Variation in mean values and SD for anxiety and depression (HADS) according to type of cancer treatment ($n=499$)

	HADS-A		HADS-D	
	Mean	SD	Mean	SD
Type of cancer treatment				
Chemotherapy (30%)	5.8	3.4	5.0	3.6
Hormonotherapy (11%)	4.4	3.5	3.1	2.8
Immunotherapy (2%)	5.3	4.5	4.3	3.9
Radiotherapy (2%)	3.8	3.3	2.5	2.9
Combination therapy (9%)	5.1	3.2	4.4	3.2
Surgery (4%)	5.9	3.2	3.5	2.4
Cancer treatment				
Yes (58%)	5.3	(4.3)	4.3	(3.4)
No (42%)	4.9	(3.5)	3.6	(3.3)
p (Kruskal-Wallis test)	0.08		0.004	

Cancer treatment and its relationship to anxiety and depression scores are presented in Table 20. Highest anxiety and depression scores were observed in patients with chemotherapy. The lowest were in patients receiving radiotherapy (only six patients). The comparison between patients who received any cancer treatment with the patients who did not showed no significant difference for the anxiety scores ($p=0.08$) but a significant difference for the depression scores ($p=0.004$).

Table 21. Pearson correlation ($n = 499$) between fatigue subscales of FAQ, fatigue intensity and its distress as measured with LASA scales of FAQ and HADS anxiety and depression scales

	Fatigue							HADS-A	HADS-D
	Last week			Last week	Last month	Last 6 months	Fatigue distress		
	Physical Mean	Affective Mean	Cognitive Mean	LASA Mean	LASA Mean	LASA Mean	LASA Mean	Mean	Mean
Fatigue (FAQ) subscales[a]									
Physical	1.0	0.39	0.49	0.71	0.61	0.44	0.59	0.40	0.53
Affective	0.39	1.0	0.26	0.31	0.26	0.22	0.31	0.61	0.44
Cognitive	0.49	0.26	1.0	0.37	0.38	0.30	0.35	0.34	0.33
Fatigue quantity (LASA)									
Last week	0.71	0.31	0.37	1.0	0.80	0.55	0.68	0.31	0.41
Last month	0.61	0.26	0.38	0.80	1.0	0.70	0.71	0.32	0.42
Last 6 months	0.44	0.22	0.30	0.55	0.70	1.0	0.66	0.31	0.34
Fatigue distress (LASA)[a]	0.59	0.31	0.35	0.68	0.71	0.66	1.0	0.41	0.43
HADS A[a]	0.40	0.61	0.34	0.31	0.32	0.31	0.41	1.0	0.66
HADS D[a]	0.53	0.44	0.33	0.41	0.42	0.34	0.43	0.66	1.0

[a] "Last week" only values measured.

Table 22. Correlation analysis of the FAQ items ($n = 499$) using Pearson correlation coefficients

	Questionnaire items	1	2	3	4	5	6	7	8	9	10	11	12	13
1	Becoming slower	1.0	0.56	0.18	0.40	0.39	0.50	0.34	0.11	0.32	0.61	0.26	0.36	0.30
2	Unusual need for rest		1.0	0.13	0.32	0.43	0.75	0.45	0.11	0.22	0.59	0.23	0.38	0.34
3	Sleeping problems at night			1.0	0.22	0.16	0.07	0.15	0.17	0.09	0.19	0.22	0.27	0.09
4	Difficulties in concentrating				1.0	0.30	0.30	0.28	0.02	0.39	0.28	0.20	0.25	0.16
5	Wish to withdraw					1.0	0.39	0.37	0.19	0.08	0.38	0.28	0.32	0.21
6	Feeling unusually tired						1.0	0.51	0.09	0.26	0.58	0.26	0.37	0.33
7	Feeling exhausted							1.0	0.19	0.11	0.36	0.30	0.33	0.29
8	Anxiety								1.0	0.01	0.11	0.23	0.12	0.03
9	Increased forgetfulness									1.0	0.23	0.10	0.17	0.17
10	Weakness										1.0	0.22	0.43	0.38
11	Feeling tense											1.0	0.27	0.16
12	Feeling unwell												1.0	0.24
13	Having heavy limbs													1.0
	Questionnaire items	14	15	15	17	18	19	20	21	22	23			
14	Experience of pleasant tiredness	1.0	0.08	−0.10	−0.05	0.01	−0.09	−0.07	−0.11	−0.02	−0.01			
15	Wish to switch off thoughts		1.0	0.05	0.21	0.12	0.17	0.15	0.20	0.27	0.20			
16	Decreased physical performance			1.0	0.30	0.11	0.29	0.67	0.59	0.18	0.38			
17	Decreased attentiveness				1.0	0.18	0.24	0.34	0.36	0.12	0.30			
18	Feeling impatient					1.0	0.18	0.13	0.20	0.26	0.13			
19	Loss of interest						1.0	0.36	0.39	0.26	0.27			
20	Loss of energy							1.0	0.65	0.23	0.38			
21	Fight overcoming inactivity								1.0	0.23	0.43			
22	Sadness									1.0	0.17			
23	Feeling sleepy during the day										1.0			

Correlations of FAQ Subscales with Fatigue Intensity, Fatigue Distress and HADS Scores

Table 21 presents the correlations of fatigue subscales with fatigue intensity, distress and HADS scores. Physical fatigue correlated more highly with quantitative fatigue of last week and last month (0.71 and 0.61) as measured with the LASA scale. Correlations with fatigue distress were less close (0.59), and those with depression were the weakest (0.53). Affective fatigue correlated most highly with anxiety (0.61) and depression (0.44) as measured with the HAD scales. Cognitive fatigue correlated moderately closely with most other variables (0.30–0.38). Quantitative fatigue of last week (LASA) was more highly correlated with fatigue of last month (0.80) than with fatigue distress (0.68). Quantitative fatigue of the last month was more highly correlated with fatigue distress (0.71) and fatigue of the last six months (0.70). Fatigue distress showed the highest correlation with quantitative fatigue of last month (0.70) and physical fatigue (0.59). There was, however, a smaller positive relationship with anxiety (0.41) and depression (0.43). Anxiety was more highly correlated with depression (0.66) and affective fatigue (0.61). Depression correlated most closely with anxiety (0.66) and with physical fatigue of last week (0.53).

Correlation Analyses Between FAQ Items

Correlation analyses between items (Table 22) with correlation coefficients above 0.50 were found for the item "becoming slower" with weakness (0.61) and unusual need for rest (0.56); for "unusual need for rest" with unusual tiredness (0.75) and weakness (0.59); for "unusual fatigue" with weakness (0.58) and feeling exhausted (0.51); for "decreased physical performance" with fighting to overcome inactivity (0.59) and loss of energy (0.67); and for "loss of energy" with fighting to overcome inactivity (0.65).

Discussion

Owing to the exploratory research approach, patient characteristics were not equally distributed in all aspects. Whereas age was equally distributed in the whole of the study population, 61% of the population were women and 39% were men. The disease was active in 36% and inactive in 64% of the patients. Almost equal numbers of the patients had and had not received anticancer treatment, but the types of treatment varied greatly. One fifth of the patients were treated as inpatients and four fifths were outpatients. The groups with different types of cancer differed considerably in size. Despite these uneven distributions of the characteristics, it has to be borne in mind that the patients with different types of cancer were categorized and some groups, such as breast cancer patients, contained only women or were associated with a uniform type of treatment. The control of most of these important variables within the disease groups accounted for the differences, and testing of the hypothesis was therefore still possible.

Psychometric Properties of the FAQ

Reliability and validity of the FAQ were tested in an earlier study in cancer patients and healthy individuals (previous chapter) and could now be supported in this wider group of cancer patients. Internal consistency for the rather short FAQ was good for the overall scale and for the physical subscale, with a Cronbach alpha coefficient of 0.90. The coefficient for the affective subscale (0.65) and the cognitive subscale (0.68) can be regarded as acceptable, considering that they include only five and three items, respectively, and that they measure subjective attributes. The overall coefficient of 0.90 supports the case for items of all the subscales measuring the same underlying latent variable (De Vellis 1990). It therefore seems reasonable to ask whether this is an argument against the division into three subscales. It can be argued, however, that physical, affective and cognitive aspects of fatigue are very much interwoven and that the validity of the multidimensional concept has been developed in qualitative research from the perspective of the patients who expressed fatigue at these three levels. The correlation coefficients of the items within the subscales further support their use.

The fatigue items of the FAQ subscales, originally generated by cancer patients and also tested in the earlier study in cancer patients and healthy individuals (previous chapter), were all again reported in similar fashion in this study population, which supports their content validity. Redundant items that did not fit into any subscale were identified by factor analysis and deleted before any further analyses, which improved the validation process further. The ability to measure differences between types and stages of cancer supports reliability and validity. The use of FAQ in this larger patient population led to the (factor-analytic) identification of three factors (Table 9), which were identified earlier, but not as clearly, in the much smaller population in the previous study (Table 6). The ability to measure differences between types and stages of cancer in this study supports reliability and validity.

The factors are now similar to those of subscales of a very recently published multidimensional fatigue inventory (Smets and Garssen 1996). This concurrently developed inventory comprises scales on general, physical and mental fatigue and on reduced activity and reduced motivation. Future research may allow testing of convergent validity of the inventory. The Piper Fatigue Scale (Piper and Lindsey 1989) also reflects a multidimensional fatigue concept but, because of its different end-points, cannot be compared with the FAQ.

The FAQ was specifically developed in and for a general cancer patient population, measuring fatigue in the physical, affective and cognitive dimensions and also measuring quantity of fatigue and the distress caused by it to include the severity dimension. It offers the possibility of identifying fatigue qualitatively at the three levels of expression and at the same time allows quantitative measurement by adding the reported items. Feasibility and acceptability have been shown to be very good. With finally 19 binary items and 2 LASA scales, it is easy to use and prevents vulnerable patients from stressful investigations. The scaling system needs to be adapted when the instrument is being used to measure changes of fatigue more sensitively (a four-point scale) rather than just epidemiologically (yes/no). The final, adapted version of FAQ, in German and in its English translation, is presented in the Appendix 1. Please note that this is not a professionally translated, validated english version.

Correlation of Fatigue with Different Types of Cancer

The investigation of fatigue in the 10 groups with different types of cancer did not reveal any significant differences between them on measurement of fatigue with the LASA scales of FAQ (Table 11). Measurement of fatigue in the same groups with the three subscales of FAQ, however, showed a significant difference for the physical subscale and a lesser degree of difference for the affective subscale (Table 10). This suggests that there is a more specific, more sensitive measurement of fatigue, with qualitative, multidimensional assessment, identifying a major discriminating physical component between types of cancer. For all cancer types, physical fatigue was most prominent, followed first by affective, and then by cognitive fatigue. Lung cancer, ovarian cancer and melanoma were associated with the highest fatigue levels. These results are in agreement with those of another study, in which high occurrence of fatigue in lung cancer patients was also confirmed (Hürny and Bernhard 1993). They also conform with observations recorded in another study, in which 59% of untreated lung cancer patients with limited disease suffered from reduced energy (Sarna 1994). Clinical experience in oncology gives the impression that lung cancer patients suffer more from fatigue than breast cancer patients. This impression has also been described by others (Smets and Garssen 1996). Gynecological cancer (without ovarian cancer), breast cancer and cancer of the testis were associated with the lowest fatigue levels. Sleep problems were far more prominent in patients with lung cancer than in other groups. Some of the groups, however, were small and therefore the results need to be interpreted with caution. It has to be added that the group of patients with breast cancer represented a much more uniform group with one type of cancer than did the group with gastrointestinal cancer, which embraced a wide variety of patients with different types of cancer, possibly with different baseline fatigue levels.

Correlation of Fatigue with Stage of Cancer

The hypothesis that fatigue correlates with stage of cancer was supported (Tables 13, 14). Again, the physical fatigue scale showed highest significance for differences between the three stages of cancer, an observation that was backed up by the LASA scale measurement for last week and last month. The increase of fatigue levels in patients with localized disease over the last six months confirmed the correlation with disease progression. It has to be considered that the group with localized disease was smaller than the other groups. The difference in levels of fatigue in the different stages may be explained either by the primary impact of growing cancer bulk on the organ system or by "asthenins" produced by the active tumor, causing asthenia (Theologides 1982). Other defense mechanisms of the body against the tumor, involving cytokines, such as TNF or interleukins, might play a part (Morant 1991). Levels of inflammatory mediators have been found to be significantly different in various tumor stages (Staal-van Brekel and Dentener 1995) in relation to weight-stable and weight-losing patients. The same could be expected in different tumor stages of specific cancer types in relation to fatigue. A study involving 1000 patients with advanced cancer, in whom the incidence of symptoms was investigated, showed that fatigue was consistently among the ten most prevalent symptoms (Donelli and Walsh 1995), which supports the correlation of fatigue with advanced stages of disease.

The distress resulting from fatigue measured in this study also progressed from cancer in remission to localized disease to metastatic disease, which underpins the relevance of the experience of fatigue. It also underlines the distressing nature of fatigue in cancer disease and differentiates it from the usual kind of tiredness perceived by healthy persons. It supports the content validity of the anchor words of the LASA scales of FAQ.

Differences Between Types and Stages in Breast Cancer, Malignant Lymphoma, and Gastrointestinal Cancer

Investigation of the different stages in beast cancer, malignant lymphoma and gastrointestinal cancer revealed a significant difference for physical fatigue in lymphoma and breast cancer patients with advanced stages of disease (Table 12). The distress caused by fatigue, however, remained significant in patients with malignant lymphoma only, which could be explained by the fact that malignant lymphomas are systemic in nature if they are active. Owing to the small numbers in the group of patients with gastrointestinal cancer, the analysis considered patients in remission versus all the rest: still no difference was found between stages in this group. As significant differences between stages of cancer in all patients had been established before, these results require further thought. It could be that some specific types of cancer, such as gastrointestinal cancers, are associated with high levels of fatigue, even in nonmetastatic states, and that these types of cancer cells excrete substances that induce fatigue even at very early stages. This would still support the hypothesis that fatigue correlates with type and stage of cancer, but it would include the hypothesis that fatigue can also correlate solely with type of cancer. Another explanation would be the presence of normal baseline fatigue levels, which do not differ at any stage. Fatigue, as measured with LASA scales for last week in gastrointestinal cancer, however, showed mean fatigue levels of 36 mm and mean fatigue distress levels of 38 mm. Mean levels of healthy individuals, as measured in the previous study in the previous chapter, were 24 mm for fatigue and 28 mm for the distress it caused (Table 8).

Disentangling Confounding Treatment Variables

The influence of anticancer treatment versus no anticancer treatment on levels of fatigue was recognizable. Significance was reached for the physical subscale, the LASA scales and for the fatigue distress scale (Table 16). These results raise the question of whether the two groups compared represent patients with active disease (receiving anticancer treatment) against patients with inactive disease (not receiving anticancer treatment). This question, however, could be answered by comparison of the patients with different stages of cancer, receiving or not receiving anticancer treatment. The fact that no significant difference was found in fatigue between anticancer treatment status in the three stages of cancer in the whole population suggests that the influence of cancer stage is more prominent than the influence of anticancer treatment. This does not exclude a fatiguing influence of anticancer treatment in otherwise nonfatigued cancer patients, such as patients with breast cancer during an adjuvant therapy. It therefore does not necessarily contradict the findings of other researchers of higher fatigue levels in women with localized breast cancer receiving a combination of radio- and chemotherapy than in those women who did not receive treatment (Woo and Dipple 1996).

However, different levels of fatigue were identified in the different treatment groups (Table 15). Chemotherapy was clearly associated with higher fatigue levels than hormone therapy or no therapy. It has to be considered that the numbers treated according to the different regimens in this study varied greatly and conclusions need to be treated with caution. A recent investigation indicated similar fatigue levels among groups receiving different chemotherapy regimens (Richardson 1996). It has to be considered that different therapy regimens usually are given to patients with different types of cancer, possibly representing different baseline fatigue levels. However, the general influence of anticancer treatment cannot be underestimated and specific types of therapy need further investigation considering longitudinal measurement in the course of treatment and also type and stage of disease.

Half of the cancer patients investigated needed some medication other than anticancer treatment. Examination of fatigue related to these non-anti-cancer medications revealed significant differences, indicating higher fatigue levels in all measurements, excluding affective fatigue, in patients who did receive such non-anti-cancer medication (Table 16). This raises the question of whether the observed difference is caused by the non-anti-cancer medication or whether the population examined represents unintended subgroups. For instance, it could be that some patients were in a curative situation whilst others were in a palliative situation, when other medications, such as analgesics, might be related to symptoms of advanced cancer. The significant occurrence of sleep problems in patients with non-anti-cancer medication might support this relationship, as sleep problems can be associated with pain, mood disturbance, or other symptoms of active disease. The significant difference between the two groups, however, needs further attention and it emphasizes the importance of controlling such variables when investigating fatigue in cancer patients.

Confounding Patient Characteristics: Age and Gender

The less significant increase found for affective fatigue in younger patients in this study supports findings of an earlier, empirical study, which reported higher emotional distress in younger patients than in older patients (Nerenz and Leventhal 1982). Results in this study showed significantly higher (physical) fatigue levels in men under the age of 50 years than in men over 50. This difference needs to be treated with caution, because women outnumbered men in the study population and the large group of women with breast cancer generally had lower fatigue levels than other disease groups. The findings that fatigue levels did not differ between women under and over the age of 50 years and between men and women generally, suggests that these characteristics are of secondary importance for the development of fatigue, as opposed to type and stage of cancer, which appear to play the primary part in this respect.

Fatigue, Anxiety, and Depression

The co-investigation of anxiety and depression in this study clearly confirmed the high correlation of anxiety and depression with stage of cancer. When the disease progressed, these emotions also increased (Table 18). The fact that depression differed significantly between all groups with different types of cancer might be related to the different prognostic outlook (Table 19). Lung cancer patients are more likely to be confronted with potentially fatal disease than are patients with cancer of the testis, and depression in lung cancer patients might be an outcome of the coping process. The same significance could be found for depression in relation to anticancer treatment; depression was higher in patients with anticancer treatment (Table 20), which could be related again to active, advancing disease needing specific treatment. The significance of depression in the group undergoing noncancer treatment might also be related to the fact that for these patients cancer-treatment was no longer available (Table 16). When anxiety and depression are compared in breast cancer, malignant lymphoma and gastrointestinal cancer patients (Table 12), it is interesting to see that patients with malignant lymphoma showed a significant difference between the stages for both anxiety and depression, but patients with gastrointestinal cancer again showed no difference for either. In breast cancer, there was a significant difference between stages concerning depression, but not for anxiety. However, when looking at levels of anxiety and depression in relation to age and gender (Table 17), all patients over the age of 50 years showed higher levels of depression (but not for anxiety) than younger patients. Men showed higher levels of depression (but not for anxiety) than women, and men over the age of 50 years showed slightly higher levels of depression (but not for anxiety) than younger men. Whereas anxiety had approximately the same influence on all the subgroups, depression was significantly focused on men over the age of 50 years in this study. As it had been shown before that there is an association of anxiety and depression with stages of cancer, further research is needed to identify further determinants. However, it could be shown that depression differed between types of cancer (Table 19), and even though the numbers between disease groups differed considerably, it can at least be stated that depression was higher in patients with lung cancer than in the other groups.

No systematic studies have yet investigated the relationship between depression and anxiety with fatigue experienced by cancer patients. Some studies have shown fatigue to be related to mood (Blesch and Paice 1991; Bruera and Brenneis 1989). Fatigue and depression could, however, also represent two completely different concepts. When the fatigue mean levels and the HADS mean levels found for the three stages in breast cancer, malignant lymphoma and gastrointestinal cancers were analyzed (Table 12), it could be said that:

1. Significantly different levels of physical fatigue between stages in patients with lymphoma were accompanied by significantly different levels of anxiety and depression.
2. The significant level of physical fatigue between stages in patients with breast cancer was accompanied by significant levels of depression (not anxiety).
3. The nonsignificance of fatigue in any measurement between stages in patients with gastrointestinal cancer was accompanied by levels of depression and anxiety that were also not significant.

The significantly higher physical fatigue levels in males at the age over 50 years (Table 17) were accompanied by significant levels of depression (not anxiety). These results strongly support a very similar concept of fatigue and depression. The only contradiction in this sense was the difference in gender. Whereas no significant difference in fatigue levels was found between male ($n=195$) and female ($n=304$) subjects generally, a significantly higher level of depression was found in men ($p=0.02$). This difference in depression could suggest that fatigue and depression are different constructs. These results need further attention.

The correlation of fatigue with depression and anxiety is of greatest interest, as the question of whether fatigue causes depression or whether depression causes fatigue is still subject to debate. The highest correlation could be seen between the affective sub scale of FAQ and anxiety of HADS (0.61) (Table 21), which indicates that anxiety is partially captured with the affective subscale in the FAQ and, to a lesser degree, also depression (0.44). A positive relationship could, however, also be observed between the physical subscale of FAQ and depression of HADS (0.53), which indicates that depression is well captured with the physical subscale in the FAQ and, to a lesser degree, also anxiety (0.40). It could be suggested that there was a trend for physical fatigue to be positively correlated with depression and affective fatigue to be positively related to anxiety. This does not explain whether they are the same experience or whether they just appear together. The relatively positive relationship between fatigue distress and depression (0.43) and anxiety (0.41) suggests a similar construct. Cognitive fatigue showed positive but less strong correlation with anxiety and depression of HADS. The tentatively proposed framework, described in the chapter "A Qualitative Exploration of the Concept of Fatigue/Tiredness in Cancer Patients and in Healthy Individuals," explaining fatigue as a multidimensional construct that is expressed at physical, affective and cognitive levels, is therefore lent further support.

Interrelationships Between Items of the FAQ

The correlation of depression with fatigue emphasized the emotional component of fatigue. Further correlation analyses of the questionnaire items supported a strong physical fatigue component. The identified descriptors with a positive relationship between them may represent components of fatigue (Table 22). It can be hypothesized that the interrelationships between these components represent the process of fatigue development. Fatigue might lead to an unusual need for rest, which in turn might lead to inactivity, weakness, and decreased physical performance, resulting in a lack of energizing metabolic resources. A vicious circle phenomenon, involving a rest/activity imbalance, has already been hypothesized in the chapters "A Qualitative Exploration of the Concept of Fatigue/Tiredness in Cancer Patients and in Healthy Individuals" and "Testing the Fatigue Assessment Questionnaire in Healthy Persons and in Cancer Patients." Further research is needed to study and test the interrelationship between these components.

Conclusions and Directions for Further Research

Reliability and validity of the new FAQ have been supported in this study with a larger cancer patient population. Factor analyses supported the theoretical framework of fatigue expression at physical, affective and cognitive levels hypothesized earlier.

There was also a correlation of stages of cancer with fatigue levels. Patients with metastatic disease generally experienced more fatigue than those in remission, although there might be types of cancer that produce high fatigue levels even in localized disease. Correlation of specific types of cancer with levels of fatigue could be confirmed to some extent. The statistical soundness of this study is limited by the variable numbers of patients in the different disease groups, but this limitation was imposed by the study's exploratory approach. Further research is needed to study patient groups of comparable size with different cancer types in order to identify further risk populations. The role of anticancer treatment has been identified as significant in this study, but it is argued that advanced stages of cancer are a major determinant factor for the development of fatigue. The role of other medications and of age and gender must be subjected to the same kind of investigation as the role of advanced disease. The importance of controlling confounding variables, such as type and stage of cancer, treatment regimen, comedication, age and gender in future fatigue research has been shown by this study.

Further research is needed to analyze the interrelationship between anxiety, depression and fatigue and between the identified components of fatigue.

References

Anderson P, Dean G (1996) A pilot test of physiological fatigue indicators in healthy controls. Abstract no 36. Annual oncology nursing congress, Philadelphia

Blesch K, Paice J (1991) Correlates of fatigue in breast or lung cancer. Oncol Nurs Forum 18:81–87

Bruera E (1988) Asthenia in patients with advanced cancer. J Pain Symptom Manage 18 (1):81–87

Bruera E, Brenneis C (1989) Association between asthenia and nutritional status, lean body mass, anemia, psychological status and tumor mass in patients with advanced breast cancer. J Pain Symptom Manage 4 (2):59–63

Butow P, Coates A (1991) On the receiving end. IV: validation of quality of life indicators. Ann Oncol 2:597–603

Chen M (1986) The epidemiology of self-perceived fatigue among adults. Prev Med 15:74–81

De Vellis R (1991) Scale development: theory and applications. Sage Publications, Newbury Park, pp 12–23; 51–90

Donelli S, Walsh D (1995) The symptoms of advanced cancer. Semin Oncol 22 [Suppl 3]:67–72

Glaus A (1993) Assessment of fatigue in cancer and non-cancer patients and in healthy individuals. J Support Care Cancer 1:305–315

Grandjean E (1968) Fatigue: its physiological and psychological significance. Ergonomics 11:427–436

Greenberg D (1990) Neurasthenia in the 1980's: chronic fatigue syndrome, anxiety and depressive disorders. Psychosomatics 31 (2):129–137

Haylock P, Hart L (1979) Fatigue in patients receiving localised radiation. Cancer Nurs 2:461–467

Herrmann C, Scholz K (1991) Psychologisches Screening von Patienten einer kardiologischen Akutklinik mit einer deutschen Fassung der Hospital Anxiety and Depression (HAD) Skala. Psychother Psychosom Med Psychol 41:83–92

Holmes S (1991) Preliminary investigation of symptom distress in two cancer patient populations: evaluation of a measurement instrument. J Adv Nurs 16:439–446

Hürny C, Bernhard J (1993) Fatigue and malaise as quality of life indicator in small-cell lung cancer patients. Support Care Cancer 1:316–320

Irvine D, Vincent L, Graydon J (1994) The prevalence and correlates of fatigue in patients receiving treatment with chemotherapy and radiotherapy. Cancer Nurs 17 (5):367–378

Karnofsky D, Abelmann W (1949) The use of the nitrogen mustards in the palliative treatment of carcinoma. Cancer 1:634–656

Keller U (1993) Pathophysiology of cancer cachexia. Support Care Cancer 1:290–294

King K, Nail L (1985) Patients' descriptions of the experience of receiving radiation therapy. Oncol Nurs Forum 12:55–61

Knoff M (1986) Physical and psychological distress associated with adjuvant chemotherapy in women with breast cancer. J Clin Oncol 4 (5):678–684

Kobashi J, Hanewald G, Van Dam F (1985) Assessment of malaise in cancer patients treated with radiotherapy. Cancer Nurs 8 (6):306–313

Koczocik J, Krzysztof B (1994) Electrophysiological studies of nerve and muscle in comparative neoplasma. Electroencephalogr Clin Neurophysiol 34:237–241

Levine PH, Atherton M (1994) An approach to studies of cancer subsequent to clusters of chronic fatigue syndrome: use of data from the Nevada State Cancer Registry. Clin Infect Dis 18 [Suppl 1]:49–53

Love R, Leventhal H (1989) Side effects and emotional distress during cancer chemotherapy. Cancer 63:604–612

McCorkle R, Young K (1978) Development of a symptom distress scale. Cancer Nurs 10:373–378

McNair D, Lorr M (1971) EITS manual for the profile f mood states. Educational and Industrial Testing Service, San Diego

Meyerowitz B, Watkins I (1983) Quality of life for breast cancer patients receiving adjuvant chemotherapy. Am J Nurs 83 (2):232–235

Morant R (1991) Asthenia in cancer patients – a double edged inflammatory response against the tumour? J Palliat Care 7:22–24

Nerenz D, Leventhal H (1982) Factors contributing to emotional distress during cancer chemotherapy. Cancer 50 (5):1020–1027

Pearson P, Byars G (1956) The development and validation of a checklist measuring subjective fatigue (report no 56–115). School of Aviation, Randolph AFB

Pickard-Holley S (1991) Fatigue in cancer patients. Cancer Nurs 14 (1):13–19

Piper B, Lindsey A (1989) Development of an instrument to measure the subjective dimension of fatigue. In: Funk S, Tournquist E (eds) Key aspects of comfort. Springer, Berlin Heidelberg New York, pp 199–280

Piper B, Rieger P (1989) Recent advances in the management of biotherapy-related side effects: fatigue. Oncol Nurs Forum [Suppl] 16 (6):27–34

Rhodes V, Watson P (1988) Patients' descriptions of the influence of tiredness and weakness on self-care abilities. Cancer Nurs 11 (3):186–194

Richardson A (1996) The experience of fatigue and other symptoms in patients receiving chemotherapy. Eur J Cancer Care 5 [Suppl 2]:24–30

Sarna L (1994) Functional status in women with lung cancer. Cancer Nurs 17 (2):87–93

Schag C, Heinrich R, Ganz P (1984) Karnofsky Performance Status Revisited: reliability, validity and guidelines. J Clin Oncol 2 (3):187–193

Smets E, Garssen B (1996) Application of the multidimensional fatigue inventory (MFI-20) in cancer patients receiving radiotherapy. Br J Cancer 73:241–245

Staal-van den Brekel A, Dentener M (1995) Increasing resting energy expenditure and weight loss are related to a systematic inflammatory response in lung cancer. J Clin Oncol 13 (10):2600–2605

Theologides A (1982) Asthenia in cancer. Am J Med 73:1–3

Winningham M, Nail L, Barton Burke M, et al (1994) Fatigue and the cancer experience: the state of the knowledge. Oncol Nurs Forum 21 (1):23–36

Woo B, Dipple L (1996) Variations in fatigue scores by treatment methods in women with breast cancer. Abstract no 182. Annual oncology nursing congress, Philadelphia

World Health Organisation (1990) Cancer pain relief and palliative care. WHO, Geneva (Technical report series 804)

Yoshitake H (1971) Relations between the symptoms and feelings of fatigue. Ergonomics 14 (1):175–186

Zigmond A, Snaith R (1983) The Hospital Anxiety and Depression Scale. Acta Psychiatr Scand 67:361–370

Synthesis and General Discussion

Study of the fatigue literature has shown tha many different concepts of fatigue have been discussed in the past and in the current century. Insofar as it concerns patients with cancer, the discussion around fatigue has become very topical in the current decade, and it is now a subject of international discussion among nurses and others engaged in research. Again, different attempts have been made to conceptualize fatigue in cancer patients (Piper and Lindsey 1989; Cimprich 1992; Irvine and Vincent 1994; Winningham and Nail 1994). This discussion will focus on the most important findings of the studies presented in this book, namely on the difference of fatigue concepts between cancer patients and healthy individuals and the importance of this difference when the use of measurement instruments is considered. Furthermore, the identification of a new concept of fatigue in cancer patients will be discussed. The relationship of a dominant physical and an affective component of fatigue with the disease will be discussed, and implications for nursing practice and research will be proposed.

Critical Design Features

Current international discussion reveals that the complexity of the concept of "fatigue" is emphasized by linguistic and cultural differences in various countries. Whereas experience shows that English-speaking nursing and medical experts assume that fatigue is a pathologic expression of otherwise healthy tiredness, some other groups, such as German, Italian or Swedish populations, realize that there is no such word as fatigue in their languages. In a German-speaking lay population, the word fatigue cannot be used because it is a foreign technical term that is only understood by health care professionals. This implies that research not only needs to define fatigue as a concept, but must also decide on its linguistic description and meaning in different languages and cultures.

The words used to describe fatigue can vary in different health conditions, apart from the differences in languages. Evidence for this was given by the results of the first study presented, which showed the linguistic differences between healthy individuals and cancer patients. Neither patients nor healthy individuals used the word "fatigue" or "malaise" in this German-speaking population when they spoke about their experience of fatigue. An important characteristic was observed in the different mood states with which the two groups described fatigue. Whereas cancer patients expressed sadness and suffering when speaking about their fatigue experience, the interviews did not put an emotional strain on healthy persons. These observations support the notion of different grounds in which fatigue feelings might be rooted for ill and healthy individuals. Sadness was unmistakably present in the fatigued cancer patients, a correlation that has been established before (Bruera 1988; Blesch and Paice 1991; Smets and Garssen 1996). In contrast, the group of healthy individuals did not appear anxious about feeling tired; they even used words that incorporated some form of humor. This observation is in accordance with statements from Nixon (1976), who described tiredness in healthy persons as a non-anxiety-inducing state. It thus becomes evident that "normal tiredness" in healthy persons and "abnormal tiredness" in cancer patients need to be differentiated.

The linguistic and cultural differences reveal only the tip of the iceberg. The whole concept of fatigue needs to be explored from the perspective of health and disease. From the perspective of physiology in health, fatigue is defined as a life-sustaining state similar to other physiological needs, such as thirst and hunger (Grandjean 1968). Grandjean, together with other authors (Dill 1967; Bartley 1967), describes fatigue as a defense mechanism, a protective phenomenon and a process of adaptation in order to maintain health. It is difficult to define the normative tiredness levels of a healthy population, however, and data taking account of gender and age are lacking. This makes it difficult to know what can be labeled as "abnormal tiredness" in diseased persons. Chen (1986) concluded in his study that 20% of healthy adults indicated that they were suffering from fatigue, which does not help to identify the level or quantity of what is considered "abnormal fatigue." Studies comparing tiredness levels of healthy individuals with those of diseased persons are lacking or show methodological difficulties, especially in terms of measurement, sample size or confounding variables (Pickard-Holley 1991; Glaus 1993).

If fatigue is to be measured quantitatively as a continuum with the aid of linear analogue scales, it becomes especially important that a valid continuum of the construct "fatigue" is defined for the population concerned. The studies presented in the chapters "A Qualitative Study to Explore the Concept of Fatigue/Tiredness in Cancer Patients and in Healthy Individuals" and "Construction of a New Fatigue Assessment Questionnaire" showed that healthy persons experience a different quality of tiredness than cancer patients. Whereas tiredness in healthy persons was mainly experienced as a pleasant consequence of hard work and was relieved by rest, cancer patients spoke about an unusual, extreme, lasting tiredness. The use of anchor words like "I do not feel tired" and "I feel very tired" fails to capture these two different types of tiredness. Symptom distress scales have not respected this difference and simply use the anchor words "I do not feel tired" and "I feel very tired" (McCorkle and Young 1978; Holmes 1991). The newly developed Fatigue Assessment Questionnaire (FAQ) took account of that differences in the linear analogue scales: words used by the cancer patients were adopted as the anchor words, and the new continuum ranked from "I did not feel unusually tired" to "I did feel extremely tired, exhausted." This difference in fatigue linear analogue scales has not been described in the literature before.

Evidence for the ability of the linear analogue scale of FAQ to distinguish between different populations was given in the study described in the chapter "Testing the Fatigue Assessment Questionnaire in Healthy Persons and in Cancer Patients." Comparison of mean fatigue levels measured with linear analogue scales between healthy individuals and cancer patients showed a significant difference ($P=0.004$): 24 mm of fatigue (for last week) in healthy persons and 38 mm for cancer patients with various cancer diagnoses. Distress caused by fatigue also remained significantly different between the two groups. The methodological implication of these results is the confirmation of sensitivity to measure the right type of fatigue in cancer patients, and the clinical implication is the availability of baseline data on quantitative fatigue in healthy individuals. Even though age and gender were equally distributed, the lack of age- and gender-adjusted subgroups could be seen as a limitation of the study. However, no such confirmatory study comparing a general cancer patient population with healthy individuals was found in the literature.

Defining a Concept of Fatigue in Cancer Patients

The literature shows that fatigue is not a new topic. In the past it has been associated with different dimensions, such as with muscle fatigue (Kronecker 1871), with mental symptoms (Cowles 1893), with "overburdening" and also with psychological aspects (MacDougall 1899). Muscio, in 1921, stated that the term fatigue should be banished from scientific discussions and that attempts to develop a fatigue test should be abandoned (Muscio 1921). This pronouncement shows that scientists working at that time had similar difficulties in defining and measuring fatigue to those we seem to have today. Not until the 1960s did fatigue become a subject for research again, when industrial research attempted to measure tiredness in airmen (Pearson and Byars 1956) and when tiredness in industrial workers became interesting in relation to working performance (Grandjean 1961; Yoshitake 1971). In the last decade, fatigue been discussed as a disease in its own right, as the "chronic fatigue syndrome," without clear evidence of its cause (Behan and Behan 1985). Today, fatigue is recognized as one of the most distressing symptoms of cancer (World Health Organisation 1990).

It has become evident that the concept of fatigue is dependent on the nature of the population to which it refers. Linguistic and cultural characteristics, health status and also the purpose of the research conducted are determining factors. This thesis aimed at identifying the concept of fatigue as it is experienced by cancer patients and it was therefore not the aim to identify causes or consequences, but the actual experiences of fatigue. Following the series of studies described in the chapters "A Qualitative Study to Explore the Concept of Fatigue/Tiredness in Cancer Patients and in Healthy Individuals," "Testing the Fatigue Assessment Questionnaire in Healthy Persons and in Cancer Patients" and "The Relationship Between Fatigue and Type and Stage of Cancer," a classification system with expression of fatigue at physical, affective and cognitive levels was identified. This new classification system led to the tentative development of a step-like theory explaining the evolution of fatigue/tiredness, which is similar to a theoretical framework described by Bruera (1994) to explain the production of pain. This theory explains the production of fatigue by involving nociception, perception and expression (see the chapter "A Qualitative Study to Explore the Concept of Fatigue/Tiredness in Cancer Patients and in Healthy Individuals"). The three studies presented in this book provide evidence that fatigue can be seen as an "umbrella term" for a multitude of components, which are expressed at the physical, affective and cognitive levels. Since it is not yet possible to identify and measure fatigue at the cortical or biochemical level, assessment has to be based on patients' subjective expressions. The basic components of physical, affective and cognitive fatigue appear to be relevant for different populations, since they were identified in both healthy individuals and cancer patients. The causes, however, appear to be different. The theoretical models described by Piper et al. (1987), Winningham and Nail (1994), and Irvine and Vincent (1994) offer a multitude of theoretical explanations for the causes and mechanisms of fatigue in patients with cancer. There is, however, no definition of the actual experience of fatigue and no measurement instrument provided for this framework.

Evidence for the concept of fatigue that has three components was first suggested in the qualitative study described in the chapter "A Qualitative Study to Explore the Concept of Fatigue/Tiredness in Cancer Patients and in Healthy Individuals," when content analysis of the unstructured interviews led to a tentative framework comprising three categories. The concept found partial agreement in the following quantitative study described in the chapter "Testing the Fatigue Assessment Questionnaire in Healthy Persons and in Cancer Patients," and it was eventually possible to confirm it in the third study, presented in the chapter "The Relationship Between Fatigue and Type and Stage of Cancer," which included a large cancer patient population. The framework, eventually derived from the factor-analytic results of the third study, explains the actual experience of fatigue in cancer patients, which is illustrated in Fig. 1. Whilst the expression of physical fatigue is dominant, the affective and cognitive expressions might be closely interwoven, and feedback mechanisms between the three levels in all directions could also be hypothesized. Further research is needed to investigate the interrelationship between these different components of fatigue.

The concept with expression of fatigue at physical, affective and cognitive levels also fitted for the healthy individuals. The content of the categories, however, has shown to be different between them. This evidence was first apparent in the study presented in the chapter "A Qualitative Study to Explore the Concept of Fatigue/Tiredness in Cancer Patients and in Healthy Indivi-

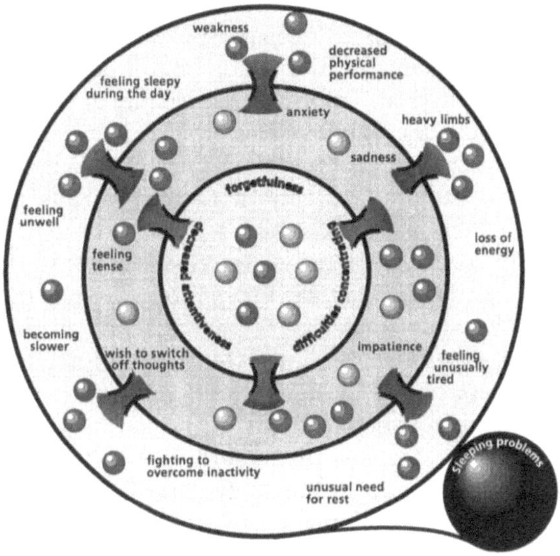

Fig. 1. The experience of fatigue in cancer patients and its expression at the physical, affective and cognitive levels

duals," where some fatigue experiences were the same in healthy persons as in cancer patients while others turned out to be very different, although fitting the same classification system. The descriptors used by healthy persons were similar to the descriptors found in the frequently used Pearson-Byars Fatigue Feeling Checklist (Pearson and Byars 1956), which was developed for the measurement of tiredness in healthy airmen, representing a continuum from "feeling peppy and refreshed" to "ready to drop." In that scale, the word fatigue is not used, which underlines its concept of "healthy tiredness." In the earlier study presented (see the chapter "A Qualitative Study to Explore the Concept of Fatigue/Tiredness in Cancer Patients and in Healthy Individuals"), circadian or even pleasant tiredness was reported by healthy individuals, and results of the consecutive study even showed an inverse correlation in cancer patients (see the chapter "Testing the Fatigue Assessment Questionnaire in Healthy Persons and in Cancer Patients"). It was suggested that a "positive or physiological type of tiredness," resulting from physical exercise or hard work, was typical for healthy individuals. However, in the third study (chapter "The Relationship Between Fatigue and Type and Stage of Cancer") with a large cancer population it could be shown that the "healthy, circadian type of tiredness" was also reported by cancer patients, indicating that they can experience more than one type of tiredness. This underlines the importance of measuring the right type of cancer-specific fatigue and the importance of using measurement instruments which include patient-centered items developed out of the population concerned. The fatigue instruments developed for healthy persons (Pearson and Byars 1956; Yoshitake 1971) and for psychological investigations (McNair and Lorr 1971) measure different types of tiredness than the cancer-specific FAQ.

Evidence for a cancer-specific type of tiredness was shown in the first study, where cancer patients spoke about the distressing type of tiredness. Their experiences had a major impact on wellbeing: expressions, such as decreased physical performance, extreme, unusual tiredness; weakness; and unusual need for rest were cancer-specific experiences and were not mentioned by healthy persons (see the chapter "A Qualitative Study to Explore the Concept of Fatigue/Tiredness in Cancer Patients and in Healthy Individuals"). One of the main differences was the occurrence of weakness in 85% of the group of cancer patients, whereas healthy individuals did not describe fatigue as weakness at all. Recent literature has recognized the need to investigate whether weakness is the same as tiredness (Winningham and Nail 1994). Data from this interview study suggest that weakness, as distinct from weakness caused by neurological damage, is an inherent part or component of fatigue in cancer patients.

Evidence for this distressing type of tiredness, possibly better called fatigue, was shown in the study described in the chapter "Testing the Fatigue Assessment Questionnaire in Healthy Persons and in Cancer Patients," which supported the qualitative analyses of fatigue with quantitative methods. Univariate analysis of the descriptors identified in the first study and then included in the new FAQ discriminated well between healthy and ill persons. Again, decreased physical performance; unusual, extreme tiredness; weakness; unusual need for rest; fight to overcome inactivity; and loss of energy were very different between healthy persons and cancer patients. At this stage, it was suggested that physical sensations of fatigue might be stronger than affective and cognitive ones, as these last two categories did not appear to discriminate between the healthy and the diseased group. Nevertheless, the less frequent occurrence of affective and cognitive sensations, overall, might also be explained by the fact that they are less tangible than the physical sensations and that patients tend to speak more openly about physical than about psychological feelings, as has been observed by other investigators (Kobashi et al. 1985). The cancer-specific fatigue descriptors, with an emphasis on the physical impact, were replicated in the third study (see the chapter "The Relationship Between Fatigue and Type and Stage of Cancer").

Throughout all three studies the physical descriptors of fatigue were more prevalent than the others. The dominant expression of physical fatigue led to a tentative hypothesis of an activity/inactivity vicious circle phenomenon (Fig. 1 in the chapter "Testing the Fatigue Assessment Questionnaire in Healthy Persons and in Cancer Patients"). The hypothesis was supported by the results of the third study (see the chapter "The Relationship Between Fatigue and Type and Stage of Cancer") in a large cancer patient population, where the same physical components were dominant with the correlation analysis showing a strong correlation between them. The hypothesis shares one aspect with Winningham's theoretical model of fatigue in cancer patients, in which fatigue is seen as a symptom caused by disease, treatment and other symptoms and as a secondary symptom of decreased activity, which leads to decreased functional status and eventually to disability (Winningham and Nail 1994). Winningham explains her fatigue theory by a lack of energizing metabolic resources, which leads to further fatigue.

The hypothesized vicious circle phenomenon partially supports the secondary fatigue caused by decreased activity explained by Winningham. It is, however, argued that important causes other than the lack of energizing metabolic resources might be involved. Fatigue, which in the vicious circle is hypothesized as the "starter" of the circle, might be caused primarily by biochemical substances, such as inflammatory mediators or cytokines, produced by different types and stages of cancer (Morant 1991; Keller 1993). The biochemical consequences of such substances might also be involved in primary and in secondary fatigue. However, fatigue might additionally be caused or at least aggravated by restricted affective and cognitive resources. Immobility, isolation and sensory deprivation have been thought to induce fatigue mechanisms that involve the inhibition of the reticular activation system (RAS) in the mid-brain and medulla, which is responsible for maintaining wakefulness and alerting the cortex. Reduced cortical activity has also been explained by chronic stimulation, such as depression, anxiety and pain (Astair 1987). These mechanisms might well be involved in secondary fatigue and might influence the activity/inactivity balance. This theory is tentative and further research is needed to substantiate it.

The third study, presented in the chapter "The Relationship Between Fatigue and Type and Stage of Cancer," has shed some light on the interrelationship between fatigue in patients with cancer and the physical and affective fatigue expression: it has become evident that physical aspects of fatigue are dominantly linked to the biochemical disease process. For example, the results showed some evidence that patients with certain types of cancer experience more fatigue than patients with other types, with lung cancer patients showing the highest fatigue levels. But these results need to be treated with caution, because the sample sizes for patients with some of the specific tumor types were probably too small (lung cancer: n=28). In comparison to those with lung cancer, patients with breast cancer (n=149) had far lower fatigue levels. The difference between types of cancer could not be statistically confirmed except with the physical subscale of FAQ. This suggests that the more qualitative measurement with the physical subscale is more sensitive than the quantitative measurement with the linear analogue scale alone. The fact that only physical fatigue differed between patients with different types of cancer and that affective and cognitive fatigue was commonly lower in patients with all cancer types supports the dominance of fatigue as a physical expression.

In the third study (see the chapter "The Relationship Between Fatigue and Type and Stage of Cancer"), quantitative fatigue levels, as measured with linear analogue scales for the period of last week, were identified in a large general cancer patient population with various diagnoses, stages and treatments (n=499). These levels were again higher than those identified earlier in healthy persons. Irvine and Vincent (1994) compared fatigue levels between healthy women and women with breast cancer and showed that there was no difference between the two groups. This strongly supports the hypothesis that there might be no differences between patients with certain types of cancer, such as breast cancer in the early stages, and healthy persons. It underscores the importance of considering type and stage of cancer in any comparison of fatigue levels in cancer patients and in healthy individuals. The difference in the sizes of cancer-specific subgroups in the third study could be responsible for the present lack of a statistically significant difference between other groups, however. Further research is needed to analyze fatigue levels more clearly in patients with specific cancer types.

The basis of the expectation that fatigue levels between different types of cancer are different is the hypothesis that the impact of cancer on the affected organ plays the primary part and that the secretion of cancer-specific "asthenins" may be a secondary cause of fatigue (Theologides 1982; Bruera 1988). A few data indicate high fatigue levels in patients with lung cancer (Blesch and Paice 1991; Butow and Coates 1991; Sarna 1994), a group of tumors known to produce more "paraendocrine" substances than other types of cancer. The influence of asthenins on energy-transformation processes and on muscle wasting have previously been discussed (Keller 1993,) but it remains unclear whether the immune system or the tumor itself is mainly responsible for their production (Morant 1991).

The correlation of fatigue with different stages of cancer was confirmed (see the chapter "The Relationship Between Fatigue and Type and Stage of Cancer"). Even the investigation of major influencing factors, such as cancer treatment, did not appear to overrule the primary association of fatigue with stage of disease. It suggests that the physical expression of fatigue is more likely to be related to the disease than to the treatment. Although radiotherapy has been shown to increase fatigue towards the end of treatment (Haylock and Hart 1979; King and Nail 1985) and although it has been demonstrated that fatigue is the most prevalent side effect in patients receiving chemotherapy and immunotherapy (Knoff 1986; Rhodes and Watson 1988; Piper and Rieger 1989; Blesch and Paice 1991; Richardson 1996), the results of that study showed that the advanced stage of cancer overruled treatment influences. This supports the theory that the stage of cancer is the major determining factor concerning development of fatigue in cancer patients, which means that the stage of cancer must be the highest priority in the search for the causal relationships. It can be concluded, therefore, that patients with advanced cancer are at higher risk of fatigue than patients with localized disease or disease in remission. This result is new and has not been investigated and reported so far.

Another important finding was that the stage of cancer was not only correlated with fatigue but also with depression and anxiety, as measured with the HADS. The same findings have been described by other researchers (Smets and Garssen 1996). This, however, does not answer the question of whether fatigue leads to depression or whether depression leads to fatigue. Data from this study indicate that fatigue in the advanced stages of cancer is highly correlated with anxiety and depression. But it was found that depression is more likely to be found in advanced stages of most cancer patients than anxiety, and that age is an important variable. It could be hypothesized that long-lasting states of anxiety over the course of chronic illness lead to exhaustion, and such anxiety was described as the forerunner of fatigue by Morris (1982). The other important message from the third study is that fatigue appears to be linked with depression in advanced cancer disease. This strongly suggests that affective fatigue might be linked to psychological coping with incurable disease. Results also suggest that treatment variables might play a part in the development of depression in advanced stages, but this needs to be interpreted with great caution because of the presence of confounding variables, such as stage and type of cancer.

The weakness of the third study (see the chapter "The Relationship Between Fatigue and Type and Stage of Cancer") is the numerical imbalance of patients in the various subgroups, which was the result of the exploratory approach of this investigation aimed at testing consecutive cancer patients in a general oncology population. Retrospectively it can be questioned whether the explorative approach of including patients with all major cancer types should have been replaced by a more controlled approach from the beginning, aimed at achieving equal numbers in defined groups. However, this would have imported considerable selection bias, and the explorative approach facilitated an interesting insight into the magnitude of the fatigue experience in a general cancer patient population with different stages of disease.

Issues for Further Research and Implications for Practice

The three subscales of the FAQ allow measurement of the physical, affective and cognitive elements of fatigue and so enable them to be correlated with other aspects of the patient and his or her disease. The inclusion of linear analogue scales for the quantitative measurement of fatigue and its distress provides insight into the relevance of the fatigue experience. This opens up the possibility of identifying more cancer-specific fatigue expression, which becomes important when the clinical effectiveness of future treatment strategies is to be assessed. The validity of the FAQ confirms the nature of the fatigue concept. In terms of internal consistency, the questionnaire has been shown to be reliable (see the chapter "The Relationship Between Fatigue and Type and Stage of Cancer"). It can be used in practice and in further research by various professionals who care for cancer patients, whether they are physicians, nurses or psychologists. For the use of FAQ in different countries, a professional translation from the German language into others is needed. The yes/no response type can be used for cross-sectional, epidemiological research. For repeated measurement over time, more finely differentiated response categories will be considered, and the use of such response categories as "not at all," "a little," "quite a bit," "very much" will be tested in the future. Any further use in research could be helpful, however, for further evaluation of the psychometric properties of the questionnaire. For the evaluation of therapeutic strategies in the care of cancer patients suffering from fatigue, reliable and validated instruments are needed to document its effectiveness.

Further research questions raised by the studies presented in this book are: (a) Is fatigue a symptom of cancer or an expression of coping with cancer? (b) Is fatigue independent of depression found in patients with advanced stages of cancer? (c) Are biochemical substances mainly responsible for physical fatigue and is psychological coping with progressive disease mainly associated with affective fatigue? (d) What is the interrelationship between the physical components of fatigue and are they responsible for a vicious circle, and if so, can it be broken?

Further research is also needed to provide definitive answers about what types of cancer are associated with the highest fatigue levels. These questions have not yet received enough attention in the literature, considering their importance for the future development of therapeutic strategies. Research will also have to deal with separating out the different causes of fatigue in cancer patients, with possible pharmacological, medical treatment and with nursing and psychological support measures.

A better understanding of the fatigue mechanisms will facilitate intervention strategies. No research has been published on the prevention of fatigue in cancer patients. This could be a focus of future clinical research, for example in patients with early stages of breast cancer receiving adjuvant treatment. Research has shown that fatigue levels in these patients correlate with the antineoplastic treatment (Woo and Dipple 1996). What kind of intervention might help these women to become less fatigued in the course of the treatment? In contrast to that, the correlations of fatigue with certain types and with advanced stage of cancer indicate a biological cause, which can be seen as an inevitable outcome of the disease (Theologides 1982). If progressive cancer cannot be influenced by treatment, it will remain difficult to prevent or treat fatigue. It then becomes a nursing and counseling challenge to help patients to understand fatigue as a symptom of disease and to support them in managing the activities of daily living with a restricted energy account. In the chapter "The Relationship Between Fatigue and Type and Stage of Cancer" it has been shown that patients with advanced cancer suffer from high fatigue levels associated with depression, which guides research and practice towards support of patients in coping in the situation of living with an incurable disease. For nurses, the hypothesis of the vicious circle of activity/inactivity might be of considerable interest, as mobilization, activity and inactivity present an important concept in nursing care. The studies have shown that any sound research methodology used in the area of fatigue requires a thorough consideration of the confounding variables, such as type and stage of cancer, treatment variables, symptom control measures, emotional status, age and gender.

A better knowledge of fatigue in cancer will not only provide the potential for therapeutically oriented research aimed at relieving fatigue, but support nurses' understanding of patients' personal fatigue experience. The increased knowledge of the caregivers will enable them to become more aware of this distressing, silent companion of many cancer patients, thus helping patients to cope with fatigue. The generation of "general fatigue knowledge" in patients with cancer should enable caregivers to deal with the expression of fatigue in a very personal way. Fatigue can also become an important area of judgement in clinical nursing practice, with fatigue measurement becoming a part of the assessment process.

It is the sincere hope of the author that the outcomes of this work will contribute both to the advancement of scientific methodology of questionnaire design and to the increase of knowledge in the domain of fatigue in cancer, thus improving individual patient care.

References

Astair J (1987) Fatigue in the cancer patients: a conceptual approach to a clinical problem. Oncol Nurs Forum 14 (6):25–30

Bartley SH (1967) The human organism as a person. Chilton, Philadelphia

Behan P, Behan W (1985) The post-viral fatigue syndrome: an analysis of the findings in 50 cases. J Infect Dis 10:211–222

Blesch K, Paice J (1991) Correlates of fatigue in people with breast or lung cancer. Oncol Nurs Forum 18 (1):81–87

Bruera E (1988) Asthenia in patients with advanced cancer. J Pain Symptom Manage 3 (1):9–13

Bruera E (1994) New developments in the assessment of pain in cancer patients. Support Care Cancer 2:312–318

Butow P, Coates A (1991) On the receiving end IV: validation of quality of life indicators. Ann Oncol 2:297–603

Chen M (1986) The epidemiology of self-perceived fatigue among adults. Prev Med 15:74–81

Cimprich B (1992) A theoretical perspective on attention and patient education. Adv Nurs Sci 14 (3):39–51

Cowles E (1893) The mental symptoms of fatigue. NY Med J 1:345–352

Dill DB (1967) The Harvard fatigue laboratory: its development contributions and demise. Circ Res 20 [Suppl 1]:161–170

Glaus A (1993) Assessment of fatigue in cancer- and non-cancer patients and in healthy individuals. Support Care Cancer 1:305–315

Grandjean E (1961) Die zentrale Ermüdung. In: Lehmann G (ed) Handbuch der gesamten Arbeitsmedizin. Urban and Schwarzenberg, Berlin, pp 442–470

Grandjean E (1968) Fatigue: its physiological and psychological significance. Ergonomics 11:427–436

Haylock P, Hart L (1979) Fatigue in patients receiving localized radiation. Cancer Nurs 2:461–467

Holmes S (1991) Preliminary investigation of symptom distress in two cancer patient populations: evaluation of a measurement instrument. J Adv Nurs 16:439–446

Irvine D, Vincent L (1994) The prevalence and correlates of fatigue in patients receiving treatment with chemotherapy and radiotherapy: a comparison with the fatigue experienced by healthy individuals. Cancer Nurs 17 (5):367–378

Keller U (1993) Pathophysiology of cancer cachexia. Support Care Cancer 1:290–294

King K, Nail L (1985) Patients descriptions of the experience of receiving radiation therapy. Oncol Nurs Forum 12:55–61

Knoff M (1986) Physical and psychological distress associated with adjuvant chemotherapy in women with breast cancer. J Clin Oncol 4 (5):678–684

Kobashi J, Hanewald G, Van Dam F (1985) Assessment of malaise in cancer patients treated with radiotherapy. Cancer Nurs 8 (6):306–313

Kronecker H (1871) Über die Ermüdung und Erholung der quergestreiften Muskeln. Ber Verh Sachs Gesell Wiss Lpg 5:710–736
MacDougall R (1899) Fatigue. Psychol Rev 6:203–208
McCorkle R, Young K (1978) Development of a symptom distress scale. Cancer Nurs 10:373–378
McNair D, Lorr M (1971) EITS manual for the profile of mood states. Educational and Industrial Testing Service, San Diego
Morant R (1991) Asthenia in cancer patients – a double-edged inflammatory response against the tumor? J Pall Care 7 (3):22–24
Morris M (1982) Tiredness and fatigue. In: Norris C (ed) Concept clarification in nursing. Aspen, Rockville, pp 263–275
Muscio B (1921) Is a fatigue test possible? Br J Psychol 12:31–46
Nixon P (1976) The human function curve. Practitioner 217:765–770
Pearson P, Byars G (1956) The development and validation of a checklist measuring subjective fatigue (report No. 56–115). School of Aviation, Randolph AFB, TX
Pickard-Holley S (1991) Fatigue in cancer patients. Cancer Nurs 14 (1):13–19
Piper B, Lindsey A (1989) Development of an instrument to measure the subjective dimension of fatigue. In: Funk S, Tournquist E (eds) Key aspects of comfort. Springer, Berlin Heidelberg New York, pp 199–280
Piper B, Rieger L (1989) Recent advances in the management of biotherapy-related side effects: fatigue. Oncol Nurs Forum 16 [Suppl 6]:27–32
Piper B, Lindsey A (1987) Fatigue mechanisms in cancer patients: developing nursing theory. Oncol Nurs Forum 14 (6):17–23
Rhodes V, Watson P (1988) Patients' descriptions of the influence of tiredness and weakness on self-care abilities. Cancer Nurs 11 (3):186–194
Richardson A (1996) Patterns of fatigue in patients receiving chemotherapy. Eur J Cancer Care [Suppl]
Sarna L (1994) Functional status in women with lung cancer. Cancer Nurs 17 (2):87–93
Smets E, Garssen B (1996) Application of the multidimensional fatigue inventory (MFI-20) in cancer patients receiving radiotherapy. Br J Cancer 73:241–245
Theologides A (1982) Asthenia in cancer. Am J Med 73:1–3
Winningham N, Nail L, Barton Burke M (1994) Fatigue and the cancer experience: the state of the knowledge. Oncol Nurs Forum 21 (1):23–36
Woo B, Dipple L (1996) Variations in fatigue scores by treatment methods in women with breast cancer. Abstract no 182. Annual oncology nursing congress, Philadelphia
World Health Organization (1990) Cancer pain relief and palliative care. WHO, Geneva (Technical report series 804)
Yoshitake H (1971) Relations between the symptoms and feelings of fatigue. Ergonomics 14 (1):175–186

Appendix

MÜDIGKEITS – FRAGEBOGEN FAQ (FATIGUE ASSESSMENT QUESTIONNAIRE), Glaus 1997 **Datum:** ______________

Code Nr. ________ Name: _______________ Vorname: ____________ Jahrgang: ______________

Bitte beantworten Sie die folgenden Fragen, indem Sie die für Sie passende Antwort einkreisen (entsprechendes einkreisen)
Die Antwort muß sich auf die Zeit der vergangenen Woche (inklusiv heute) beziehen

	überhaupt nicht	wenig	mäßig	sehr
1. Reagierten, handelten Sie langsamer?	1	2	3	4
2. Verspürten Sie ein extremes, unübliches Bedürfnis, sich auszuruhen? (unüblich für Sie)	1	2	3	4
3. Verspürten Sie ein Gefühl extremer, unüblicher Müdigkeit? (unüblich für Sie)	1	2	3	4
4. Erlebten Sie ein Gefühl von „ausgewunden sein", von Erschöpfung?	1	2	3	4
5. Verspürten Sie eine Schwäche, einen Verlust an Kraft?	1	2	3	4
6. Verspürten Sie ein allgemeines Unwohlgefühl?	1	2	3	4
7. Verspürten Sie schwere Glieder?	1	2	3	4
8. Verspürten Sie eine reduzierte, körperliche Leistungsfähigkeit?	1	2	3	4
9. Verspürten Sie einen Verlust an Energie? (verglichen mit Ihrer üblichen Energie)	1	2	3	4
10. Brauchte es oft Überwindung, die sonst üblichen Aktivitäten durchzuführen?	1	2	3	4
11. Fühlten Sie sich während des Tages oft schläfrig?	1	2	3	4
12. Hatten Sie Schwierigkeiten, sich zu konzentrieren?	1	2	3	4
13. Fühlten Sie sich vergesslicher als normalerweise?	1	2	3	4
14. War es für Sie schwierig, aufmerksam zu bleiben, zum Beispiel beim Zuhören oder Lesen?	1	2	3	4
15. Hatten Sie den Wunsch, die Gedanken „abzuschalten"?	1	2	3	4
16. Verspürten Sie Angst?	1	2	3	4
17. Fühlten Sie sich angespannt?	1	2	3	4
18. Fühlten Sie sich ungeduldig?	1	2	3	4
19. Fühlten Sie sich traurig, deprimiert?	1	2	3	4
20. Hatten Sie nachts Schlafprobleme?	1	2	3	4

Auf der nächsten Seite folgen noch weitere Fragen dazu, wie intensiv Sie die unübliche Müdigkeit letzte Woche und letzten Monat empfunden und wie stark Sie darunter gelitten haben.

Auf der Vorderseite zeigen wir Ihnen zuerst, wie Sie die Fragen beantworten können.

ZUERST EIN BEISPIEL DAS IHNEN ZEIGT, WIE SIE DIE SKALEN AUSFÜLLEN KÖNNEN

Wenn Sie sich beispielsweise in der vergangenen Woche extrem stark, unüblich müde gefühlt haben, jedoch nicht komplett erschöpft waren, würden Sie einen Strich auf die Linie setzen wie folgt:

Ich fühlte mich überhaupt nicht unüblich müde	*Beispiel* ______________________________	Ich fühlte mich extrem müde komplett erschöpft

Den Strich ganz links auf die Linie zu setzen bedeutet, daß Sie überhaupt nicht unüblich müde waren. Je weiter Sie den Strich nach rechts setzen, desto mehr Müdigkeit geben Sie an. Wenn Sie den Strich ganz rechts setzen, bedeutet das, daß Sie extrem müde, komplett erschöpft waren.
Nun beantworten Sie bitte noch die letzten Fragen in dieser Weise auf der Rückseite dieses Formulars. Besten Dank.

Code Nr. ______ Name/Vorname: ______________________________

Wie stark fühlten Sie sich unüblich müde? (Unüblich bedeutet ungewöhnlich für Sie)

Bitte setzten Sie einen geraden Strich dort auf die Linie, wo es der Müdigkeit, die Sie empfunden haben, am ehesten entspricht.

a) in der letzten Woche	Ich fühlte mich überhaupt nicht unüblich müde	______________________________	Ich fühlte mich extrem müde total erschöpft
b) im letzten Monat	Ich fühlte mich überhaupt nicht unüblich müde	______________________________	Ich fühlte mich extrem müde total erschöpft

c) Wenn Sie sich in einer dieser Zeitspannen unüblich müde fühlten, wie stark litten Sie unter dieser Müdigkeit ?

Ich litt überhaupt nicht darunter	______________________________	Ich litt sehr stark darunter

Hilfe beim Ausfüllen:
- ja
- nein

FATIGUE ASSESSMENT QUESTIONNAIRE (FAQ), Glaus 1997 **Date:** ______________

Code Nr. ______ Name: ______________________________ year of birth: _________

Please answer the following questions by circling the number which indicates best which was correct for you.
During past week.

	Not at all	A little	Quite a bit	Very much
1. Did you become slower in doing, reacting?	1	2	3	4
2. Did you experience an extreme, unusual need for rest (unusual for you)	1	2	3	4
3. Did you experience a feeling of extreme, unusual tiredness (unusual for you)?	1	2	3	4
4. Did you experience a feeling of being worn out, of exhaustion?	1	2	3	4
5. Did you experience weakness, loss of strength?	1	2	3	4
6. Did you experience a feeling of general unwellness?	1	2	3	4
7. Did you experience heavy limbs?	1	2	3	4
8. Have you experienced decreased, physical performance?	1	2	3	4
9. Did you experience a loss of energy (compared to your usual energy)?	1	2	3	4
10. Did you experience the need to force yourself to do things, to overcomeinactivity?	1	2	3	4
11. Did you often feel sleepy during day-time?	1	2	3	4
12. Did you experience difficulties in concentrating?	1	2	3	4
13. Did you feel more forgetful than usual?	1	2	3	4
14. Did you find it difficult to be attentive (e.g. for listening, reading)?	1	2	3	4
15. Did you experience the wish to "switch off" the thoughts?	1	2	3	4
16. Did you experience anxiety?	1	2	3	4
17. Did you feel tense?	1	2	3	4
18. Did you feel impatient?	1	2	3	4
19. Did you feel sad?	1	2	3	4
20. Did you experience sleeping problems (at night)?	1	2	3	4

On the following page follow further questions on how intensively you experienced unusual tiredness during last week and during last month and how much distress this caused to you.

Not translated professionally yet into the English language.

Here we first show you how you can answer the questions.

FIRST AN EXAMPLE HOW YOU CAN ANSWER THE QUESTIONS

If you, for example, felt unusual, extreme tiredness last week, but did not feel completely exhausted, you would put a mark on the scale as the example shows:

I did not feel unusually tired at all.	*Example* ______________________	I felt extremely tired exhausted

To put the mark at the very left side on the line would indicate, that you did not experience any unusual tiredness. The more you put the mark on the right side on the line, the more you indicate that you felt unusually tired. To put the mark at the very right side on the line, means that you felt extremely tired, exhausted.
Now please answer the questions on the back page of this paper. Thank you.

Code Nr. ______ Name: __________________ Date: ____________

How much unusual tiredness did you experience? (unusual for you, extremely tired)

Please set a mark on the line were it best describes the unusual tiredness which you experienced

a) Last week	I did not feel unusually tired at all	______________________________	I felt extremely tired, exhausted
b) Last month	I did not feel unusually tired at all	______________________________	I felt extremely tired, exhausted

c) If you felt unusually tired in one of these periods, how much have you been distressed by this tiredness?

I was not distressed by it at all	______________________________	I was very much distressed by it

Subject Index